*God Is in
the Manger*

DIETRICH BONHOEFFER

God Is in the Manger

Reflections on Advent and Christmas

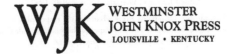

TRANSLATED BY O. C. DEAN JR.

COMPILED AND EDITED BY JANA RIESS

WJK WESTMINSTER
JOHN KNOX PRESS
LOUISVILLE · KENTUCKY

© 2010 Westminster John Knox Press

First edition
Published by Westminster John Knox Press
Louisville, Kentucky

10 11 12 13 14 15 16 17 18 19—10 9 8 7 6 5 4 3 2 1

Scripture quotations from the New Revised Standard Version of the Bible are copyright © 1989 by the Division of Christian Education of the National Council of the Churches of Christ in the U.S.A. and are used by permission.

Scripture quotations from the Revised Standard Version of the Bible are copyright © 1946, 1952, 1971, and 1973 by the Division of Christian Education of the National Council of the Churches of Christ in the U.S.A. and are used by permission.

Devotional text herein originally appeared in
Dietrich Bonhoeffer's *I Want to Live These Days with You: A Year of Daily Devotions* (Louisville, KY: Westminster John Knox Press, 2007).

Book design by Drew Stevens
Cover design by designpointinc.com

Library of Congress Cataloging-in-Publication Data

Bonhoeffer, Dietrich, 1906–1945.
  [Selections. English. 2010]
  God is in the manger : reflections on Advent and Christmas / by Dietrich Bonhoeffer ; translated by O. C. Dean Jr. ; compiled and edited by Jana Riess. —1st ed.
    p. cm.
  Includes bibliographical references and index.
  ISBN 978-0-664-23429-4 (alk. paper)
  1. Advent—Meditations. 2. Christmas—Meditations I. Riess, Jana. II. Title.
  BV40.B66513 2010
  242'.33—dc22

                                                          2010003667

PRINTED IN THE UNITED STATES OF AMERICA

CONTENTS

TRANSLATOR'S PREFACE

Since Dietrich Bonhoeffer wrote before the days of inclusive gender, his works reflect a male-oriented world in which, for example, the German words for "human being" and "God" are masculine, and male gender was understood as common gender. In this respect, his language has, for the most part, been updated in accordance with the practices of the New Revised Standard Version of the Bible (NRSV); that is, most references to human beings have become gender-inclusive, whereas references to the Deity have remained masculine.

While scriptural quotations are mostly from the NRSV, it was necessary at times to substitute the King James Version (KJV), the Revised Standard Version (RSV), or a literal translation of Luther's German version, as quoted by Bonhoeffer, in order to allow the author to make his point. In a few other cases, the translation was adjusted to reflect the wording of the NRSV.

O. C. Dean Jr.

EDITOR'S PREFACE

⸺ ⟨∞⟩ ⸺

This devotional brings together daily reflections from one of the twentieth century's most beloved theologians, Dietrich Bonhoeffer (1906–1945). These reflections have been chosen especially for the seasons of Advent and Christmas, a time when the liturgical calendar highlights several themes of Bonhoeffer's beliefs and teachings: that Christ expresses strength best through weakness, that faith is more important than the beguiling trappings of religion, and that God is often heard most clearly by those in poverty and distress.[1]

Although he came from a well-to-do family, by the time he wrote most of the content in this book, Bonhoeffer was well acquainted with both poverty and distress. Just two days after Adolf Hitler had seized control of Germany in early 1933, Bonhoeffer delivered a radio sermon in which he criticized the new regime and warned Germans that "the Führer concept" was dangerous and wrong. "Leaders of offices which set themselves up as gods mock God," his address concluded. But Germany never got to hear those final statements, because Bonhoeffer's microphone had been switched off mid-transmission.[2] This began a twelve-year struggle against Nazism in Germany, with Bonhoeffer running afoul of authorities and being arrested in 1943. Much of the content of this book was written during the two years he spent in prison.

For Bonhoeffer, waiting—one of the central themes of the Advent experience—was a fact of life during the war: waiting to be released from prison; waiting to be able to spend more than an hour a month in the company of his young fiancée, Maria von Wedemeyer; waiting for the end of the war. In his absence, friends and former students were killed in battle and his parents' home was bombed; there was little he could do about any of this except pray and wield a powerful pen. There was a helplessness in his situation that he recognized as a parallel to Advent, Christians' time of waiting for redemption in Christ. "Life in a prison cell may well be compared to Advent," Bonhoeffer wrote his best friend Eberhard Bethge as the holidays approached in 1943. "One waits, hopes, and does this, that, or the other—things that are really of no consequence—the door is shut, and can only be opened *from the outside*."[3]

But the prison door was never opened for Bonhoeffer, not in life at least. As the Third Reich crumbled in April 1945, Hitler ordered the execution of some political prisoners who had conspired to overthrow him. Since papers had recently been discovered that confirmed Bonhoeffer's involvement in this anti-Nazi plot, the theologian was among those scheduled to be executed in one of Hitler's final executive decrees.[4] Bonhoeffer was hanged on April 8, 1945, just ten days before German forces began to surrender and less than three weeks before Hitler's own death by suicide. Bonhoeffer was just thirty-nine years old.

Although Bonhoeffer's death (and the narrow timing of it) is tragic, we are fortunate that he was a prolific writer who left behind so many lectures, papers, letters, and diary entries from which we may piece together his theology.

HOW TO USE THIS BOOK

Advent is rarely exactly four weeks long, and can in fact vary in length from year to year. It always begins four Sundays before Christmas (December 25), but since Christmas falls on a different day of the week each year, Advent can begin anywhere between November 27 on the early side and December 3 on the late side. The first four weeks of this devotional assume the earliest possible start date, so that if Advent falls on or around November 27, you will have four full weeks of devotions to see you through to Christmas Day. If you're using the book in a year when Advent is slightly shorter, feel free to skip a few devotions in the first or last week.

The four Advent weeks are arranged by theme — waiting, mystery, redemption, and incarnation — and are followed by devotions for the twelve days of Christmas, which stretch from Christmas Day until January 5, just before the liturgical feast of Epiphany. These last entries are dated, since the twelve days of Christmas always begin on December 25 and end on January 5, unlike the varying days of Advent. This book also includes a final reflection for January 6, the feast of Epiphany.

Each day's devotion has a reflection from Dietrich Bonhoeffer, a Scripture to contemplate, and some bonus material. Most of the latter material is drawn from Bonhoeffer's own letters, sermons, and poetry, showing how he celebrated Christmas even when imprisoned and separated from family and beloved friends. It's important to remember how Bonhoeffer's beliefs were forged in the crucible of war and protest, and did not simply fall from the sky; it's equally important to recognize how intimately connected he was to those he loved. He did not exist in a vacuum. His legacy has also been profound, so a few of the bonus entries are taken from thinkers who might be called "heirs of Bonhoeffer"—contemporary Christian writers like Eugene Peterson, Luci Shaw, and Frederica Mathewes-Green, who reflect on some of the same issues that he did.

WAITING

The Advent Season Is a Season of Waiting

Jesus stands at the door knocking (Rev. 3:20). In total reality, he comes in the form of the beggar, of the dissolute human child in ragged clothes, asking for help. He confronts you in every person that you meet. As long as there are people, Christ will walk the earth as your neighbor, as the one through whom God calls you, speaks to you, makes demands on you. That is the great seriousness and great blessedness of the Advent message. Christ is standing at the door; he lives in the form of a human being among us. Do you want to close the door or open it?

It may strike us as strange to see Christ in such a near face, but he said it, and those who withdraw from the serious reality of the Advent message cannot talk of the coming of Christ in their heart, either. . . .

Christ is knocking. It's still not Christmas, but it's also still not the great last Advent, the last coming of Christ. Through all the Advents of our life that we celebrate runs the longing for the last Advent, when the word will be: "See, I am making all things new" (Rev. 21:5).

The Advent season is a season of waiting, but our whole life is an Advent season, that is, a season of waiting for the last Advent, for the time when there will be a new heaven and a new earth.

❖   ❖   ❖

We can, and should also, celebrate Christmas despite the ruins around us. . . . I think of you as you now sit together with the children and with all the Advent decorations — as in earlier years you did with us. We must do all this, even more intensively because we do not know how much longer we have.[1]

Letter to Bonhoeffer's parents, November 29, 1943, written from Tegel prison camp

Listen! I am standing at the door, knocking; if you hear my voice and open the door, I will come in to you and eat with you, and you with me.

Revelation 3:20

Waiting Is an Art

Celebrating Advent means being able to wait. Waiting is an art that our impatient age has forgotten. It wants to break open the ripe fruit when it has hardly finished planting the shoot. But all too often the greedy eyes are only deceived; the fruit that seemed so precious is still green on the inside, and disrespectful hands ungratefully toss aside what has so disappointed them. Whoever does not know the austere blessedness of waiting—that is, of hopefully doing without—will never experience the full blessing of fulfillment.

Those who do not know how it feels to struggle anxiously with the deepest questions of life, of their life, and to patiently look forward with anticipation until the truth is revealed, cannot even dream of the splendor of the moment in which clarity is illuminated for them. And for those who do not want to win the friendship and love of another person—who do not expectantly open up their soul to the soul of the other person, until friendship and love come, until they make their entrance—for such people the deepest blessing of the one life of two intertwined souls will remain forever hidden.

For the greatest, most profound, tenderest things in the world, we must wait. It happens not here in a storm but according to the divine laws of sprouting, growing, and becoming.

Be brave for my sake, dearest Maria, even if this letter is your only token of my love this Christmas-tide. We shall both experience a few dark hours — why should we disguise that from each other? We shall ponder the incomprehensibility of our lot and be assailed by the question of why, over and above the darkness already enshrouding humanity, we should be subjected to the bitter anguish of a separation whose purpose we fail to understand. . . . And then, just when everything is bearing down on us to such an extent that we can scarcely withstand it, the Christmas message comes to tell us that all our ideas are wrong, and that what we take to be evil and dark is really good and light because it comes from God. Our eyes are at fault, that is all. God is in the manger, wealth in poverty, light in darkness, succor in abandonment. No evil can befall us; whatever men may do to us, they cannot but serve the God who is secretly revealed as love and rules the world and our lives.[2]

Letter to fiancée Maria von Wedemeyer
from prison, December 13, 1943

A shoot shall come out from the stump of Jesse,
    and a branch shall grow out of his roots.
The spirit of the LORD shall rest on him,
    the spirit of wisdom and understanding,
    the spirit of counsel and might,
    the spirit of knowledge and the fear of the LORD.
His delight shall be in the fear of the LORD.

He shall not judge by what his eyes see,
    or decide by what his ears hear;
but with righteousness he shall judge the poor.
                                    Isaiah 11:1–4a

Not Everyone Can Wait

Not everyone can wait: neither the sated nor the satisfied nor those without respect can wait. The only ones who can wait are people who carry restlessness around with them and people who look up with reverence to the greatest in the world. Thus Advent can be celebrated only by those whose souls give them no peace, who know that they are poor and incomplete, and who sense something of the greatness that is supposed to come, before which they can only bow in humble timidity, waiting until he inclines himself toward us—the Holy One himself, God in the child in the manger. God is coming; the Lord Jesus is coming; Christmas is coming. Rejoice, O Christendom!

I think we're going to have an exceptionally good Christmas. The very fact that every outward circumstance precludes our making provision for it will show whether we can be content with what is truly essential. I used to be very fond of thinking up and buying presents, but now that we have nothing to give, the gift God gave us in the birth of Christ will seem all the more glorious; the emptier our hands, the better we understand what Luther meant by his dying words: "We're beggars; it's true." The poorer our quarters, the more clearly we perceive that our hearts should be Christ's home on earth.[3]

Letter to fiancée Maria von Wedemeyer,
December 1, 1943

Then he looked up at his disciples and said:
"Blessed are you who are poor,
for yours is the kingdom of God.
"Blessed are you who are hungry now,
for you will be filled.
"Blessed are you who weep now,
for you will laugh.
"Blessed are you when people hate you, and when they exclude you, revile you, and defame you on account of the Son of Man. Rejoice in that day and leap for joy, for surely your reward is great in heaven; for that is what their ancestors did to the prophets.
"But woe to you who are rich,
for you have received your consolation.
"Woe to you who are full now,
for you will be hungry.
"Woe to you who are laughing now,
for you will mourn and weep.
"Woe to you when all speak well of you, for that is what their ancestors did to the false prophets."

Luke 6:20–26

An Un-Christmas-Like Idea

When the old Christendom spoke of the coming again of the Lord Jesus, it always thought first of all of a great day of judgment. And as un-Christmas-like as this idea may appear to us, it comes from early Christianity and must be taken with utter seriousness. . . . The coming of God is truly not only a joyous message, but is, first, frightful news for anyone who has a conscience. And only when we have felt the frightfulness of the matter can we know the incomparable favor. God comes in the midst of evil, in the midst of death, and judges the evil in us and in the world. And in judging it, he loves us, he purifies us, he sanctifies us, he comes to us with his grace and love. He makes us happy as only children can be happy.

We have become so accustomed to the idea of divine love and of God's coming at Christmas that we no longer feel the shiver of fear that God's coming should arouse in us. We are indifferent to the message, taking only the pleasant and agreeable out of it and forgetting the serious aspect, that the God of the world draws near to the people of our little earth and lays claim to us.[4]

Dietrich Bonhoeffer, "The Coming
of Jesus in Our Midst"

❖ ❖ ❖

In that region there were shepherds living in the fields, keeping watch over their flock by night. Then an angel of the Lord stood before them, and the glory of the Lord shone around them, and they were terrified. But the angel said to them, "Do not be afraid; for see — I am bringing you good news of great joy for all the people: to you is born this day in the city of David a Savior, who is the Messiah, the Lord. This will be a sign for you: you will find a child wrapped in bands of cloth and lying in a manger." And suddenly there was with the angel a multitude of the heavenly host, praising God and saying,

> "Glory to God in the highest heaven,
>   and on earth peace among those whom
>   he favors!"

Luke 2:8–14

A Soft, Mysterious Voice

In the midst of the deepest guilt and distress of the people, a voice speaks that is soft and mysterious but full of the blessed certainty of salvation through the birth of a divine child (Isa. 9:6–7). It is still seven hundred years until the time of fulfillment, but the prophet is so deeply immersed in God's thought and counsel that he speaks of the future as if he saw it already, and he speaks of the salvific hour as if he already stood in adoration before the manger of Jesus. "For a child has been born for us." What will happen one day is already real and certain in God's eyes, and it will be not only for the salvation of future generations but already for the prophet who sees it coming and for his generation, indeed, for all generations on earth. "For a child has been born *for us*." No human spirit can talk like this on its own. How are we who do not know what will happen next year supposed to understand that someone can look forward many centuries? And the times then were no more transparent than they are today. Only the Spirit of God, who encompasses the beginning and end of the world, can in such a way reveal to a chosen person the mystery of the future, so that he must prophesy for strengthening believers and warning unbelievers. This individual voice ultimately enters into the nocturnal adoration of the shepherds (Luke 2:15–20) and into the full jubilation of the Christ-believing community: "For a child has been born for us, a son given to us."

❖ ❖ ❖

A shaking of heads, perhaps even an evil laugh, must go through our old, smart, experienced, self-assured world, when it hears the call of salvation of believing Christians: "For a child has been born for us, a son given to us."[5]

Dietrich Bonhoeffer

❖ ❖ ❖

For a child has been born for us,
    a son given to us;
authority rests upon his shoulders;
    and he is named
Wonderful Counselor, Mighty God,
    Everlasting Father, Prince of Peace.
His authority shall grow continually,
    and there shall be endless peace
for the throne of David and his kingdom.
    He will establish and uphold it
with justice and with righteousness
    from this time onward and forevermore.
The zeal of the LORD of hosts will do this.

Isaiah 9:6–7

Silence: Waiting for God's Word

We are silent in the early hours of each day, because God is supposed to have the first word, and we are silent before going to sleep, because to God also belongs the last word. We are silent solely for the sake of the word, not in order to show dishonor to the word but in order to honor and receive it properly. Silence ultimately means nothing but waiting for God's word and coming away blessed by God's word.... Silence before the word, however, will have its effect on the whole day. If we have learned to be silent before the word, we will also learn to be economical with silence and speech throughout the day. There is an impermissible self-satisfied, prideful, offensive silence. This teaches us that what is important is never silence in itself. The silence of the Christian is a listening silence, a humble silence that for the sake of humility can also be broken at any time. It is a silence in connection with the word. . . . In being quiet there is a miraculous power of clarification, of purification, of bringing together what is important. This is a purely profane fact. Silence before the word, however, leads to the right hearing and thus also to the right speaking of the word of God at the right time. A lot that is unnecessary remains unsaid.

❖   ❖   ❖

Today is Remembrance Sunday. Will you have a memorial service for B. Riemer? It would be nice, but difficult. Then comes Advent, with all its happy memories for us. It was you who really opened up to me the world of music-making that we have carried on during the weeks of Advent. Life in a prison cell may well be compared to Advent: one waits, hopes, and does this, that, or the other—things that are really of no consequence—the door is shut, and can only be opened *from the outside.*[6]

Letter from Bonhoeffer at Tegel prison to
Eberhard Bethge, November 21, 1943

❖   ❖   ❖

For God alone my soul waits in silence,
    for my hope is from him.
He alone is my rock and my salvation,
    my fortress; I shall not be shaken.
On God rests my deliverance and my honor;
    my mighty rock, my refuge is in God.
Trust in him at all times, O people;
    pour out your heart before him;
    God is a refuge for us.

Psalm 62:5–8

God's Holy Present

Serve the opportune time." The most profound matter will be revealed to us only when we consider that not only does the world have its time and its hours, but also that our own life has its time and its hour of God, and that behind these times of our lives traces of God become visible, that under our paths are the deepest shafts of eternity, and every step brings back a quiet echo from eternity. It is only a matter of understanding the deep, pure form of these times and representing them in our conduct of life. Then in the middle of our time we will also encounter God's holy present. "My times are in your hand" (Ps. 31:15). Serve your times, God's present in your life. God has sanctified your time. Every time, rightly understood, is immediate to God, and God wants us to be fully what we are. . . . Only those who stand with both feet on the earth, who are and remain totally children of earth, who undertake no hopeless attempts at flight to unreachable heights, who are content with what they have and hold on to it thankfully—only they have the full power of the humanity that serves the opportune time and thus eternity. . . . The Lord of the ages is God. The turning point of the ages is Christ. The right spirit of the ages is the Holy Spirit.

❖   ❖   ❖

Dear parents . . . I don't need to tell you how much I long for freedom and for you all. But over the decades you have provided for us such incomparably beautiful Christmases that my thankful remembrance of them is strong enough to light up one dark Christmas. Only such times can really reveal what it means to have a past and an inner heritage that is independent of chance and the changing of the times. The awareness of a spiritual tradition that reaches through the centuries gives one a certain feeling of security in the face of all transitory difficulties. I believe that those who know they possess such reserves of strength do not need to be ashamed even of softer feelings—which in my opinion are still among the better and nobler feelings of humankind—when remembrance of a good and rich past calls them forth. Such feelings will not overwhelm those who hold fast to the values that no one can take from them.[7]

Letter to Bonhoeffer's parents, written from
Tegel prison, December 17, 1943

For I hear the whispering of many—
    terror all around!—
as they scheme together against me,
    as they plot to take my life.

But I trust in you, O LORD;
    I say, "You are my God."
My times are in your hand;
    deliver me from the hand of my enemies
        and persecutors.
Let your face shine upon your servant;
    save me in your steadfast love.

Psalm 31:13–16

MYSTERY

Respect for the Mystery

The lack of mystery in our modern life is our downfall and our poverty. A human life is worth as much as the respect it holds for the mystery. We retain the child in us to the extent that we honor the mystery. Therefore, children have open, wide-awake eyes, because they know that they are surrounded by the mystery. They are not yet finished with this world; they still don't know how to struggle along and avoid the mystery, as we do. We destroy the mystery because we sense that here we reach the boundary of our being, because we want to be lord over everything and have it at our disposal, and that's just what we cannot do with the mystery. . . . Living without mystery means knowing nothing of the mystery of our own life, nothing of the mystery of another person, nothing of the mystery of the world; it means passing over our own hidden qualities and those of others and the world. It means remaining on the surface, taking the world seriously only to the extent that it can be *calculated* and *exploited*, and not going beyond the world of calculation and exploitation. Living without mystery means not seeing the crucial processes of life at all and even denying them.

❖ ❖ ❖

Ascension joy—inwardly we must become very quiet to hear the soft sound of this phrase at all. Joy lives in its quietness and incomprehensibility. This joy is in fact incomprehensible, for the comprehensible never makes for joy.[1]

Dietrich Bonhoeffer

❖　❖　❖

I want their hearts to be encouraged and united in love, so that they may have all the riches of assured understanding and have the knowledge of God's mystery, that is, Christ himself, in whom are hidden all the treasures of wisdom and knowledge.

Colossians 2:2–3

The Mystery of Love

The mystery remains a mystery. It withdraws from our grasp. Mystery, however, does not mean simply not knowing something.

The greatest mystery is not the most distant star; on the contrary, the closer something comes to us and the better we know it, then the more mysterious it becomes for us. The greatest mystery to us is not the most distant person, but the one next to us. The mystery of other people is not reduced by getting to know more and more about them. Rather, in their closeness they become more and more mysterious. And the final depth of all mystery is when two people come so close to each other that they *love* each other. Nowhere in the world does one feel the might of the mysterious and its wonder as strongly as here. When two people know everything about each other, the mystery of the love between them becomes infinitely great. And only in this love do they understand each other, know everything about each other, know each other completely. And yet, the more they love each other and know about each other in love, the more deeply they know the mystery of their love. Thus, knowledge about each other does not remove the mystery, but rather makes it more profound. *The very fact* that the other person is so near to me is the greatest mystery.

❖　❖　❖

All that is Christmas originates in heaven and comes from there to us all, to you and me alike, and forms a stronger bond between us than we could ever forge by ourselves.[2]

Maria von Wedemeyer to Dietrich Bonhoeffer,
December 19, 1943, from Pätzig

❖ ❖ ❖

I thank my God every time I remember you, constantly praying with joy in every one of my prayers for all of you, because of your sharing in the gospel from the first day until now. I am confident of this, that the one who began a good work among you will bring it to completion by the day of Jesus Christ. It is right for me to think this way about all of you, because you hold me in your heart, for all of you share in God's grace with me, both in my imprisonment and in the defense and confirmation of the gospel. For God is my witness, how I long for all of you with the compassion of Christ Jesus. And this is my prayer, that your love may overflow more and more with knowledge and full insight to help you to determine what is best, so that in the day of Christ you may be pure and blameless, having produced the harvest of righteousness that comes through Jesus Christ for the glory and praise of God. I want you to know, beloved, that what has happened to me has actually helped to spread the gospel, so that it has become known throughout the whole imperial guard and to everyone else that my imprisonment is for Christ; and most of the brothers and sisters, having been made confident in the Lord by my imprisonment, dare to speak the word with greater boldness and without fear.

Philippians 1:3–14

The Wonder of All Wonders

God travels wonderful ways with human beings, but he does not comply with the views and opinions of people. God does not go the way that people want to prescribe for him; rather, his way is beyond all comprehension, free and self-determined beyond all proof.

Where reason is indignant, where our nature rebels, where our piety anxiously keeps us away: that is precisely where God loves to be. There he confounds the reason of the reasonable; there he aggravates our nature, our piety—that is where he wants to be, and no one can keep him from it. Only the humble believe him and rejoice that God is so free and so marvelous that he does wonders where people despair, that he takes what is little and lowly and makes it marvelous. And that is the wonder of all wonders, that God loves the lowly. . . . God is not ashamed of the lowliness of human beings. God marches right in. He chooses people as his instruments and performs his wonders where one would least expect them. God is near to lowliness; he loves the lost, the neglected, the unseemly, the excluded, the weak and broken.

❖ ❖ ❖

That . . . is the unrecognized mystery of this world: Jesus Christ. That this Jesus of Nazareth, the carpenter, was himself the Lord of glory: that was the mystery of God. It was a mystery because God became poor, low, lowly, and weak out of love for humankind, because God became a human being like us, so that we would become divine, and because he came to us so that we would come to him. God as the one who becomes low for our sakes, *God in Jesus of Nazareth—that is the secret, hidden wisdom* . . . that "no eye has seen nor ear heard nor the human heart conceived" (1 Cor. 2:9). . . . That is the *depth of the Deity,* whom *we worship as mystery* and *comprehend as mystery.*[3]

Dietrich Bonhoeffer

❖ ❖ ❖

None of the rulers of this age understood this; for if they had, they would not have crucified the Lord of glory. But, as it is written,

"What no eye has seen, nor ear heard,
    nor the human heart conceived,
what God has prepared for those who love
        him"—

these things God has revealed to us through the Spirit; for the Spirit searches everything, even the depths of God.

1 Corinthians 2:8–10

The Scandal of Pious People

The lowly God-man is the scandal of pious people and of people in general. This scandal is his historical ambiguity. The most incomprehensible thing for the pious is this man's claim that he is not only a pious human being but also the Son of God. Whence his authority: "But I say to you" (Matt. 5:22) and "Your sins are forgiven" (Matt. 9:2). If Jesus' nature had been deified, this claim would have been accepted. If he had given signs, as was demanded of him, they would have believed him. But at the point where it really mattered, he held back. And that created the scandal. Yet everything depends on this fact. If he had answered the Christ question addressed to him through a miracle, then the statement would no longer be true that he became a human being like us, for then there would have been an exception at the decisive point. . . . If Christ had documented himself with miracles, we would naturally believe, but then Christ would not be our salvation, for then there would not be faith in the God who became human, but only the recognition of an alleged supernatural fact. But that is not faith. . . . Only when I forgo visible proof, do I believe in God.

❖   ❖   ❖

The kingdom belongs to people who aren't trying to look good or impress anybody, even themselves. They are not plotting how they can call attention to themselves, worrying about how their actions will be interpreted or wondering if they will get gold stars for their behavior. Twenty centuries later, Jesus speaks pointedly to the preening ascetic trapped in the fatal narcissism of spiritual perfectionism, to those of us caught up in boasting about our victories in the vineyard, to those of us fretting and flapping about our human weaknesses and character defects. The child doesn't have to struggle to get himself in a good position for having a relationship with God; he doesn't have to craft ingenious ways of explaining his position to Jesus; he doesn't have to create a pretty face for himself; he doesn't have to achieve any state of spiritual feeling or intellectual understanding. All he has to do is happily accept the cookies, the gift of the kingdom.[4]

Brennan Manning, *The Ragamuffin Gospel*

But we proclaim Christ crucified, a stumbling block to Jews and foolishness to Gentiles, but to those who are the called, both Jews and Greeks, Christ the power of God and the wisdom of God. For God's foolishness is wiser than human wisdom, and God's weakness is stronger than human strength.

1 Corinthians 1:23–25

The Power and Glory of the Manger

For the great and powerful of this world, there are only two places in which their courage fails them, of which they are afraid deep down in their souls, from which they shy away. These are the manger and the cross of Jesus Christ. No powerful person dares to approach the manger, and this even includes King Herod. For this is where thrones shake, the mighty fall, the prominent perish, because God is with the lowly. Here the rich come to nothing, because God is with the poor and hungry, but the rich and satisfied he sends away empty. Before Mary, the maid, before the manger of Christ, before God in lowliness, the powerful come to naught; they have no right, no hope; they are judged. . . .

❖ ❖ ❖

Who among us will celebrate Christmas correctly? Whoever finally lays down all power, all honor, all reputation, all vanity, all arrogance, all individualism beside the manger; whoever remains lowly and lets God alone be high; whoever looks at the child in the manger and sees the glory of God precisely in his lowliness.[5]

Dietrich Bonhoeffer

And Mary said,
"My soul magnifies the Lord,
  and my spirit rejoices in God my Savior,
for he has looked with favor on the lowliness of his
      servant.
  Surely, from now on all generations will call me
  blessed;
for the Mighty One has done great things for me,
  and holy is his name.
His mercy is for those who fear him
  from generation to generation.
He has shown strength with his arm;
  he has scattered the proud in the thoughts of
      their hearts.
He has brought down the powerful from their
      thrones,
  and lifted up the lowly;
he has filled the hungry with good things,
  and sent the rich away empty.
He has helped his servant Israel,
  in remembrance of his mercy,
  according to the promise he made to our
      ancestors,
  to Abraham and to his descendants forever."

Luke 1:46–55

The Mysteries of God

No priest, no theologian stood at the manger of Bethlehem. And yet all Christian theology has its origin in the wonder of all wonders: that God became human. Holy theology arises from knees bent before the mystery of the divine child in the stable. Without the holy night, there is no theology. "God is revealed in flesh," the God-human Jesus Christ—that is the holy mystery that theology came into being to protect and preserve. How we fail to understand when we think that the task of theology is to solve the mystery of God, to drag it down to the flat, ordinary wisdom of human experience and reason! Its sole office is to preserve the miracle as miracle, to comprehend, defend, and glorify God's mystery precisely as mystery. This and nothing else, therefore, is what the early church meant when, with never flagging zeal, it dealt with the mystery of the Trinity and the person of Jesus Christ. . . . If Christmas time cannot ignite within us again something like a love for holy theology, so that we—captured and compelled by the wonder of the manger of the Son of God—must reverently reflect on the mysteries of God, then it must be that the glow of the divine mysteries has also been extinguished in our heart and has died out.

❖   ❖   ❖

Wonder is the only adequate launching pad for exploring this fullness, this wholeness, of human life. Once a year, each Christmas, for a few days at least, we and millions of our neighbors turn aside from our preoccupations with life reduced to biology or economics or psychology and join together in a community of wonder. The wonder keeps us open-eyed, expectant, alive to life that is always more than we can account for, that always exceeds our calculations, that is always beyond anything we can make.[6]

Eugene Peterson

When the angels had left them and gone into heaven, the shepherds said to one another, "Let us go now to Bethlehem and see this thing that has taken place, which the Lord has made known to us." So they went with haste and found Mary and Joseph, and the child lying in the manger. When they saw this, they made known what had been told them about this child; and all who heard it were amazed at what the shepherds told them. But Mary treasured all these words and pondered them in her heart. The shepherds returned, glorifying and praising God for all they had heard and seen, as it had been told them.

Luke 2:15–20

An Unfathomable Mystery

In an incomprehensible reversal of all righteous and pious thinking, God declares himself guilty to the world and thereby extinguishes the guilt of the world. God himself takes the humiliating path of reconciliation and thereby sets the world free. God wants to be guilty of our guilt and takes upon himself the punishment and suffering that this guilt brought to us. God stands in for godlessness, love stands in for hate, the Holy One for the sinner. Now there is no longer any godlessness, any hate, any sin that God has not taken upon himself, suffered, and atoned for. Now there is no more reality and no more world that is not reconciled with God and in peace. That is what God did in his beloved Son Jesus Christ. *Ecce homo*—see the incarnate God, the unfathomable mystery of the love of God for the world. God loves human beings. God loves the world—not ideal human beings but people as they are, not an ideal world but the real world.

We prepare to witness a mystery. More to the point, we prepare to witness *the* Mystery, the *God made flesh*. While it is good that we seek to know the Holy One, it is probably not so good to presume that we ever complete the task, to suppose that we ever know anything about him except what he has *made known* to us. The prophet Isaiah helps us to remember our limitations when he writes, "To whom then will you compare me . . . ? says the Holy One. . . ." Think of it like this: he cannot be exhausted by our ideas about him, but he is everywhere suggested. He cannot be comprehended, but he can be touched. His coming in the flesh—this Mystery we prepare to glimpse again—confirms that he is to be touched.[7]

Scott Cairns, in *God with Us*

❖ ❖ ❖

To whom then will you liken God,
 or what likeness compare with him? . . .
. . . .
Have you not known? Have you not heard?
  Has it not been told you from the beginning?
  Have you not understood from the foundations of
    the earth?
It is he who sits above the circle of the earth,
  and its inhabitants are like grasshoppers;
who stretches out the heavens like a curtain,
  and spreads them like a tent to live in;
who brings princes to naught,
  and makes the rulers of the earth as nothing.

Isaiah 40:18, 21–23

REDEMPTION

Jesus Enters into the Guilt of Human Beings

Jesus does not want to be the only perfect human being at the expense of humankind. He does not want, as the only guiltless one, to ignore a humanity that is being destroyed by its guilt; he does not want some kind of human ideal to triumph over the ruins of a wrecked humanity. Love for real people leads into the fellowship of human guilt. Jesus does not want to exonerate himself from the guilt in which the people he loves are living. A love that left people alone in their guilt would not have real people as its object. So, in vicarious responsibility for people and in his love for real human beings, Jesus becomes the one burdened by guilt—indeed, the one upon whom all human guilt ultimately falls and the one who does not turn it away but bears it humbly and in eternal love. As the one who acts responsibly in the historical existence of humankind, as the human being who has entered reality, Jesus becomes guilty. But because his historical existence, his incarnation, has its sole basis in God's love for human beings, it is the love of God that makes Jesus become guilty. Out of selfless love for human beings, Jesus leaves his state as the one without sin and enters into the guilt of human beings. He takes it upon himself.

❖　❖　❖

We have something to hide. We have secrets, worries, thoughts, hopes, desires, passions which no one else gets to know. We are sensitive when people get near those domains with their questions. And now, against all rules of tact the Bible speaks of the truth that in the end we will appear before Christ with everything we are and were. . . . And we all know that we could justify ourselves before any human court, but not before this one. Lord, who can justify themselves?[1]

Bonhoeffer's sermon for Repentance
Sunday, November 19, 1933

❖　❖　❖

For all of us must appear before the judgment seat of Christ, so that each may receive recompense for what has been done in the body, whether good or evil.

2 Corinthians 5:10

Taking on Guilt

Because what is at stake for Jesus is not the proclamation and realization of new ethical ideals, and thus also not his own goodness (Matt. 19:17), but solely his love for real human beings, he can enter into the communication of their guilt; he can be loaded down with their guilt. . . . It is his love alone that lets him become guilty. Out of his selfless love, out of his sinless nature, Jesus enters into the guilt of human beings; he takes it upon himself. A sinless nature and guilt bearing are bound together in him indissolubly. As the sinless one Jesus takes guilt upon himself, and under the burden of this guilt, he shows that he is the sinless one.

Lord Jesus, come yourself, and dwell with us, be human as we are, and overcome what overwhelms us. Come into the midst of my evil, come close to my unfaithfulness. Share my sin, which I hate and which I cannot leave. Be my brother, Thou Holy God. Be my brother in the kingdom of evil and suffering and death.[2]

Sermon for Advent Sunday,
December 2, 1928

❖ ❖ ❖

Then someone came to him and said, "Teacher, what good deed must I do to have eternal life?" And he said to him, "Why do you ask me about what is good? There is only one who is good. If you wish to enter into life, keep the commandments." He said to him, "Which ones?" And Jesus said, "You shall not murder; You shall not commit adultery; You shall not steal; You shall not bear false witness; Honor your father and mother; also, You shall love your neighbor as yourself."

Matthew 19:16–19

Becoming Guilty

Because Jesus took upon himself the guilt of all people, everyone who acts responsibly becomes guilty. Those who want to extract themselves from the responsibility for this guilt, also remove themselves from the ultimate reality of human existence. Moreover, they also remove themselves from the redeeming mystery of the sinless guilt bearing of Jesus Christ and have no share in the divine justification that covers this event. They place their personal innocence above their responsibility for humankind, and they are blind to the unhealed guilt that they load on themselves in this very way. They are also blind to the fact that real innocence is revealed in the very fact that for the sake of other people it enters into the communion of their guilt. Through Jesus Christ, the nature of responsible action includes the idea that the sinless, the selflessly loving become the guilty.

❖　❖　❖

In eight days, we shall celebrate Christmas and now for once let us make it really a festival of Christ in our world. . . . . It is not a light thing to God that every year we celebrate Christmas and do not take it seriously. His word holds and is certain. When he comes in his glory and power into the world in the manger, he will put down the mighty from their seats, unless ultimately, ultimately they repent.[3]

Sermon to a London church on the third
Sunday of Advent, December 17, 1933

❖ ❖ ❖

Come now, let us argue it out,
    says the LORD:
though your sins are like scarlet,
    they shall be like snow;
though they are red like crimson,
    they shall become like wool.
Isaiah 1:18

Look Up, Your Redemption
Is Drawing Near

Let's not deceive ourselves. "Your redemption is drawing near" (Luke 21:28), whether we know it or not, and the only question is: Are we going to let it come to us too, or are we going to resist it? Are we going to join in this movement that comes down from heaven to earth, or are we going to close ourselves off? Christmas is coming—whether it is with us or without us depends on each and every one of us.

Such a true Advent happening now creates something different from the anxious, petty, depressed, feeble Christian spirit that we see again and again, and that again and again wants to make Christianity contemptible. This becomes clear from the two powerful commands that introduce our text: "Look up and raise your heads" (Luke 21:28 RSV). Advent creates people, new people. We too are supposed to become new people in Advent. Look up, you whose gaze is fixed on this earth, who are spellbound by the little events and changes on the face of the earth. Look up to these words, you who have turned away from heaven disappointed. Look up, you whose eyes are heavy with tears and who are heavy and who are crying over the fact that the earth has gracelessly torn us away. Look up, you who, burdened with guilt, cannot lift your eyes. Look up, your redemption is drawing near. Something different from what you see daily will happen. Just be aware, be watchful, wait just another short moment. Wait and something quite new will break over you: God will come.

❖ ❖ ❖

You know what a mine disaster is. In recent weeks we have had to read about one in the newspapers.

The moment even the most courageous miner has dreaded his whole life long is here. It is no use running into the walls; the silence all around him remains. . . . The way out for him is blocked. He knows the people up there are working feverishly to reach the miners who are buried alive. Perhaps someone will be rescued, but here in the last shaft? An agonizing period of waiting and dying is all that remains.

But suddenly a noise that sounds like tapping and breaking in the rock can be heard. Unexpectedly, voices cry out, "Where are you, help is on the way!" Then the disheartened miner picks himself up, his heart leaps, he shouts, "Here I am, come on through and help me! I'll hold out until you come! Just come soon!" A final, desperate hammer blow to his ear, now the rescue is near, just one more step and he is free.

We have spoken of Advent itself. That is how it is with the coming of Christ: "Look up and raise your heads, because your redemption is drawing near."[4]

Bonhoeffer's Advent sermon in a London
church, December 3, 1933

❖ ❖ ❖

Now when these things begin to take place, stand up and raise your heads, because your redemption is drawing near.

Luke 21:28

World Judgment and World Redemption

When God chooses Mary as the means when God himself wants to come into the world in the manger of Bethlehem, this is not an idyllic family affair. It is instead the beginning of a complete reversal, a new ordering of all things on this earth. If we want to participate in this Advent and Christmas event, we cannot simply sit there like spectators in a theater and enjoy all the friendly pictures. Rather, we must join in the action that is taking place and be drawn into this reversal of all things ourselves. Here we too must act on the stage, for here the spectator is always a person acting in the drama. We cannot remove ourselves from the action.

With whom, then, are we acting? Pious shepherds who are on their knees? Kings who bring their gifts? What is going on here, where Mary becomes the mother of God, where God comes into the world in the lowliness of the manger? World judgment and world redemption—that is what's happening here. And it is the Christ child in the manger himself who holds world judgment and world redemption. He pushes back the high and mighty; he overturns the thrones of the powerful; he humbles the haughty; his arm exercises power over all the high and mighty; he lifts what is lowly, and makes it great and glorious in his mercy.

❖ ❖ ❖

Close to you I waken in the dead of night,
And start with fear — are you lost to me once more?
    Is it always vainly that I seek you, you, my past?
I stretch my hands out,
and I pray —
and a new thing now I hear;
"The past will come to you once more,
and be your life's enduring part,
through thanks and repentance.
Feel in the past God's deliverance and goodness,
Pray him to keep you today and tomorrow."[5]

Poem written in Tegel prison, 1944

"For God so loved the world that he gave his only Son, so that everyone who believes in him may not perish but may have eternal life.

"Indeed, God did not send the Son into the world to condemn the world, but in order that the world might be saved through him. Those who believe in him are not condemned; but those who do not believe are condemned already, because they have not believed in the name of the only Son of God. And this is the judgment, that the light has come into the world, and people loved darkness rather than light because their deeds were evil. For all who do evil hate the light and do not come to the light, so that their deeds may not be exposed. But those who do what is true come to the light, so that it may be clearly seen that their deeds have been done in God."

John 3:16–21

Overcoming Fear

Human beings are dehumanized by fear. . . . But they should not be afraid. We should not be afraid! That is the difference between human beings and the rest of creation, that in all hopelessness, uncertainty, and guilt, they know a hope, and this hope is: Thy will be done. Yes. Thy will be done. . . . We call the name of the One before whom the evil in us cringes, before whom fear and anxiety must themselves be afraid, before whom they shake and take flight; the name of the One who alone conquered fear, captured it and led it away in a victory parade, nailed it to the cross and banished it to nothingness; the name of the One who is the victory cry of the humanity that is redeemed from the fear of death—Jesus Christ, the one who was crucified and lives. He alone is the Lord of fear; it knows him as its Lord and yields to him alone. Therefore, look to him in your fear. Think about him, place him before your eyes, and call him. Pray to him and believe that he is now with you and helps you. The fear will yield and fade, and you will become free through faith in the strong and living Savior Jesus Christ (Matt. 8:23–27).

❖ ❖ ❖

Only when we have felt the terror of the matter, can we recognize the incomparable kindness. God comes into the very midst of evil and death, and judges the evil in us and in the world. And by judging us, God cleanses and sanctifies us, comes to us with grace and love. . . . God wants to always be with us, wherever we may be—in our sin, suffering, and death. We are no longer alone; God is with us.[6]

"The Coming of Jesus in Our Midst"

❖ ❖ ❖

And when he got into the boat, his disciples followed him. A windstorm arose on the sea, so great that the boat was being swamped by the waves; but he was asleep. And they went and woke him up, saying, "Lord, save us! We are perishing!" And he said to them, "Why are you afraid, you of little faith?" Then he got up and rebuked the winds and the sea; and there was a dead calm. They were amazed, saying, "What sort of man is this, that even the winds and the sea obey him?"

Matthew 8:23–27

God Does Not Want to Frighten People

The Bible never wants to make us fearful. God does not want people to be afraid—not even of the last judgment. Rather, he wants to let human beings know everything, so that they will know all about life and its meaning. He lets people know even today, so that they may already live their lives openly and in the light of the last judgment. He lets us know solely for one reason: so that we may find the way to Jesus Christ, so that we may turn away from our evil way and try to find him, Jesus Christ. God does not want to frighten people. He sends us the word of judgment only so that we will reach all the more passionately, all the more avidly, for the promise of grace, so that we will know that we cannot prevail before God on our own strength, that before him we would have to pass away, but that in spite of everything he does not want our death, but our life. . . . Christ judges, that is, grace is judge and forgiveness and love—whoever clings to it is already set free.

Repentance means turning away from one's own work to the mercy of God. The whole Bible calls to us and cheers us: Turn back, turn back! Return—where to? To the everlasting grace of God, who does not leave us. . . . God will be merciful—so come, judgment day! Lord Jesus, make us ready. We rejoice. Amen.[7]

Bonhoeffer's sermon for Repentance
Sunday, November 19, 1933

❖   ❖   ❖

From that time Jesus began to proclaim, "Repent, for the kingdom of heaven has come near."

Matthew 4:17

INCARNATION

God Becomes Human

God becomes human, really human. While we endeavor to grow out of our humanity, to leave our human nature behind us, God becomes human, and we must recognize that God wants us also to become human—really human. Whereas we distinguish between the godly and the godless, the good and the evil, the noble and the common, God loves real human beings without distinction. . . . God takes the side of real human beings and the real world against all their accusers. . . . But it's not enough to say that God takes care of human beings. This sentence rests on something infinitely deeper and more impenetrable, namely, that in the conception and birth of Jesus Christ, God took on humanity in bodily fashion. God raised his love for human beings above every reproach of falsehood and doubt and uncertainty by himself entering into the life of human beings as a human being, by bodily taking upon himself and bearing the nature, essence, guilt, and suffering of human beings. Out of love for human beings, God becomes a human being. He does not seek out the most perfect human being in order to unite with that person. Rather, he takes on human nature as it is.

❖   ❖   ❖

This is about the birth of a child, not of the astonishing work of a strong man, not of the bold discovery of a wise man, not of the pious work of a saint. It really is beyond all our understanding: the birth of a child shall bring about the great change, shall bring to all mankind salvation and deliverance.[1]

"The Government upon the Shoulders of a Child," Christmas 1940

❖   ❖   ❖

In the beginning was the Word, and the Word was with God, and the Word was God. He was in the beginning with God. All things came into being through him, and without him not one thing came into being. What has come into being in him was life, and the life was the light of all people. The light shines in the darkness, and the darkness did not overcome it.

John 1:1–5

Human Beings Become Human
Because God Became Human

The figure of Jesus Christ takes shape in human beings. Human beings do not take on an independent form of their own. Rather, what gives them form and maintains them in their new form is always and only the figure of Jesus Christ himself. It is therefore not an imitation, not a repetition of his form, but their own form that takes shape in human beings. Human beings are not transformed into a form that is foreign to them, not into the form of God, but into their own form, a form that belongs to them and is essential to them. Human beings become human because God became human, but human beings do not become God. They could not and cannot bring about that change in their form, but God himself changes his form into human form, so that human beings—though not becoming God—can become human.

In Christ the form of human beings before God was created anew. It was not a matter of place, of time, of climate, of race, of the individual, of society, of religion, or of taste, but rather a question of the life of humanity itself that it recognized in Christ its image and its hope. What happened to Christ happened to humanity.

❖   ❖   ❖

The whole Christian story is strange. Frederick Buechner describes the Incarnation as "a kind of vast joke whereby the creator of the ends of the earth comes among us in diapers." He concludes, "Until we too have taken the idea of the God-man seriously enough to be scandalized by it, we have not taken it as seriously as it demands to be taken."

But we have taken the idea as seriously as a child can. America is far from spiritually monolithic, but the vast backdrop of our culture is Christian, and for most of us it is the earliest faith we know. The "idea of the God-man" is not strange or scandalous, because it first swam in milk and butter on the top of our oatmeal decades ago. At that age, many things were strange, though most were more immediately palpable. A God-filled baby in a pile of straw was a pleasant image, but somewhat theoretical compared with the heart-stopping exhilaration of a visit from Santa Claus. The way a thunderstorm ripped the night sky, the hurtling power of the automobile Daddy drove so bravely, the rapture of ice cream—how could the distant Incarnation compete with those?

We grew up with the Jesus story, until we outgrew it. The last day we walked out of Sunday School may be the last day we seriously engaged this faith.[2]

Frederica Mathewes-Green,
At the Corner of East and Now

❖   ❖   ❖

When I was a child, I spoke like a child, I thought like a child, I reasoned like a child; when I became an adult, I put an end to childish ways. For now we see in a mirror, dimly, but then we will see face to face. Now I know only in part; then I will know fully, even as I have been fully known.

1 Corinthians 13:11–12

Christmas, Fulfilled Promise

Moses died on the mountain from which he was permitted to view from a distance the promised land (Deut. 32:48–52). When the Bible speaks of God's promises, it's a matter of life and death. . . . The language that reports this ancient history is clear. Anyone who has seen God must die; the sinner dies before the promise of God. Let's understand what that means for us so close to Christmas. The great promise of God—a promise that is infinitely more important than the promise of the promised land—is supposed to be fulfilled at Christmas. . . . The Bible is full of the proclamation that the great miracle has happened as an act of God, without any human doing. . . . What happened? God had seen the misery of the world and had come himself in order to help. Now he was there, not as a mighty one, but in the obscurity of humanity, where there is sinfulness, weakness, wretchedness, and misery in the world. That is where God goes, and there he lets himself be found by everyone. And this proclamation moves through the world anew, year after year, and again this year also comes to us.

We all come with different personal feelings to the Christmas festival. One comes with pure joy as he looks forward to this day of rejoicing, of friendships renewed, and of love. . . . Others look for a moment of peace under the

Christmas tree, peace from the pressures of daily work. . . . Others again approach Christmas with great apprehension. It will be no festival of joy to them. Personal sorrow is painful especially on this day for those whose loneliness is deepened at Christmastime. . . . And despite it all, Christmas comes. Whether we wish it or not, whether we are sure or not, we must hear the words once again: Christ the Savior is here! The world that Christ comes to save is our fallen and lost world. None other.[3]

Sermon to a German-speaking church in
Havana, Cuba, December 21, 1930

❖ ❖ ❖

In the sixth month the angel Gabriel was sent by God to a town in Galilee called Nazareth, to a virgin engaged to a man whose name was Joseph, of the house of David. The virgin's name was Mary. And he came to her and said, "Greetings, favored one! The Lord is with you." But she was much perplexed by his words and pondered what sort of greeting this might be. The angel said to her, "Do not be afraid, Mary, for you have found favor with God. And now, you will conceive in your womb and bear a son, and you will name him Jesus. He will be great, and will be called the Son of the Most High, and the Lord God will give to him the throne of his ancestor David. He will reign over the house of Jacob forever, and of his kingdom there will be no end."

Luke 1:26–33

The Great Turning Point of All Things

What kings and leaders of nations, philosophers and artists, founders of religions and teachers of morals have tried in vain to do—that now happens through a newborn child. Putting to shame the most powerful human efforts and accomplishments, a child is placed here at the midpoint of world history—a child born of human beings, a son given by God (Isa. 9:6). That is the mystery of the redemption of the world; everything past and everything future is encompassed here. The infinite mercy of the almighty God comes to us, descends to us in the form of a child, his Son. That this child is born *for us*, this son is given *to us*, that this human child and Son of God belongs to me, that I know him, have him, love him, that I am his and he is mine—on this alone my life now depends. A child has our life in his hands. . . .

❖　❖　❖

How shall we deal with such a child? Have our hands, soiled with daily toil, become too hard and too proud to fold in prayer at the sight of this child? Has our head become too full of serious thoughts . . . that we cannot bow our head in humility at the wonder of this child? Can we not forget all our stress and struggles, our sense of importance, and for once worship the child, as did the shepherds and the wise men from the East, bowing before the divine child in the manger like children?[4]

"The Government upon the Shoulders
of the Child," Christmas 1940

❖   ❖   ❖

What then are we to say about these things? If God is for us, who is against us? He who did not withhold his own Son, but gave him up for all of us, will he not with him also give us everything else? Who will bring any charge against God's elect? It is God who justifies. Who is to condemn? It is Christ Jesus, who died, yes, who was raised, who is at the right hand of God, who indeed intercedes for us.

Romans 8:31–34

God Became a Child

Mighty God" (Isa. 9:6) is the name of this child. The child in the manger is none other than God himself. Nothing greater can be said: God became a child. In the Jesus child of Mary lives the almighty God. Wait a minute! Don't speak; stop thinking! Stand still before this statement! God became a child! Here he is, poor like us, miserable and helpless like us, a person of flesh and blood like us, our brother. And yet he is God; he is might. Where is the divinity, where is the might of the child? In the divine love in which he became like us. His poverty in the manger is his might. In the might of love he overcomes the chasm between God and humankind, he overcomes sin and death, he forgives sin and awakens from the dead. Kneel down before this miserable manger, before this child of poor people, and repeat in faith the stammering words of the prophet: "Mighty God!" And he will be your God and your might.

But now it is true that in three days, Christmas will come once again. The great transformation will once again happen. God would have it so. Out of the waiting, hoping, longing world, a world will come in which the promise is given. All crying will be stilled. No tears shall flow. No lonely sorrow shall afflict us anymore, or threaten.[5]

Sermon to a German-speaking church in
Havana, Cuba, December 21, 1930

And the Word became flesh and lived among us, and we have seen his glory, the glory as of a father's only son, full of grace and truth.

John 1:14

The Unfathomably Wise Counselor

Wonderful Counselor" (Isa. 9:6) is the name of this child. In him the wonder of all wonders has taken place; the birth of the Savior-child has gone forth from God's eternal counsel. In the form of a human child, God gave us his Son; God became human, the Word became flesh (John 1:14). That is the wonder of the love of God for us, and it is the unfathomably wise Counselor who wins us this love and saves us. But because this child of God is his own Wonderful Counselor, he himself is also the source of all wonder and all counsel. To those who recognize in Jesus the wonder of the Son of God, every one of his words and deeds becomes a wonder; they find in him the last, most profound, most helpful counsel for all needs and questions. Yes, before the child can open his lips, he is full of wonder and full of counsel. Go to the child in the manger. Believe him to be the Son of God, and you will find in him wonder upon wonder, counsel upon counsel.

❖ ❖ ❖

In winter it seems that the season of Spring will never come, and in both Advent and Lent it's the waiting that's hard, the in-between of divine promise and its fulfillment. . . . Most of us find ourselves dangling in this hiatus, which in the interval may seem a waste of time. . . . But "the longer we wait, the larger we become, and the more joyful our expectancy." With such motivation, we can wait as we sense that God is indeed *with us*, and at work within us, as he was with Mary as the Child within her grew.[6]

Poet Luci Shaw, in *God with Us*

But when the fullness of time had come, God sent his Son, born of a woman, born under the law, in order to redeem those who were under the law, so that we might receive adoption as children. And because you are children, God has sent the Spirit of his Son into our hearts, crying, "Abba! Father!" So you are no longer a slave but a child, and if a child then also an heir, through God.

Galatians 4:4–7

The One Who Became Human

Who is this God? This God is the one who became human as we became human. He is completely human. Therefore, nothing human is foreign to him. The human being that I am, Jesus Christ was also. About this human being Jesus Christ we say: this one is God. This does not mean that we already knew beforehand who God is. Nor does it mean that the statement "this human being is God" adds anything to being human. God and human being are not thought of as belonging together through a concept of nature. The statement "this human being is God" is meant entirely differently. The divinity of this human being is not something additional to the human nature of Jesus Christ. The statement "this human being is God" *is the vertical from above*, the statement that applies to Jesus Christ the human being, which neither adds anything nor takes anything away, but qualifies the whole human being as God. . . . Faith is ignited from Jesus Christ the human being. . . . If Jesus Christ is to be described as God, then we do not speak of his omnipotence and omniscience, but of his cradle and his cross. There is no "divine being" as omnipotence, as omnipresence.

❖ ❖ ❖

And now Christmas is coming and you won't be there. We shall be apart, yes, but very close together. My thoughts will come to you and accompany you. We shall sing "Friede auf Erden" [Peace on Earth] and pray together, but we shall sing "Ehre sei Gott in der Höhe!" [Glory be to God on high] even louder. That is what I pray for you and for all of us, that the Savior may throw open the gates of heaven for us at darkest night on Christmas Eve, so that we can be joyful in spite of everything.[7]

> Maria von Wedemeyer to Bonhoeffer,
> December 10, 1943

❖   ❖   ❖

In those days a decree went out from Emperor Augustus that all the world should be registered. This was the first registration and was taken while Quirinius was governor of Syria. All went to their own towns to be registered. Joseph also went from the town of Nazareth in Galilee to Judea, to the city of David called Bethlehem, because he was descended from the house and family of David. He went to be registered with Mary, to whom he was engaged and who was expecting a child. While they were there, the time came for her to deliver her child. And she gave birth to her firstborn son and wrapped him in bands of cloth, and laid him in a manger, because there was no place for them in the inn.

Luke 2:1–7

THE TWELVE
DAYS OF
CHRISTMAS
AND EPIPHANY

Living by God's Mercy

We cannot approach the manger of the Christ child in the same way we approach the cradle of another child. Rather, when we go to his manger, something happens, and we cannot leave it again unless we have been judged or redeemed. Here we must either collapse or know the mercy of God directed toward us.

What does that mean? Isn't all of this just a way of speaking? Isn't it just pastoral exaggeration of a pretty and pious legend? What does it mean that such things are said about the Christ child? Those who want to take it as a way of speaking will do so and continue to celebrate Advent and Christmas as before, with pagan indifference. For us it is not just a way of speaking. For that's just it: it is God himself, the Lord and Creator of all things, who is so small here, who is hidden here in the corner, who enters into the plainness of the world, who meets us in the help- lessness and defenselessness of a child, and wants to be with us. And he does this not out of playfulness or sport, because we find that so touching, but in order to show us where he is and who he is, and in order from this place to judge and devalue and dethrone all human ambition.

The throne of God in the world is not on human thrones, but in human depths, in the manger. Stand- ing around his throne there are no flattering vassals but dark, unknown, questionable figures who cannot get their fill of this miracle and want to live entirely by the mercy of God.

"Joy to the world!" Anyone for whom this sound is foreign, or who hears in it nothing but weak enthusiasm, has not yet really heard the gospel. For the sake of humankind, Jesus Christ became a human being in a stable in Bethlehem: Rejoice, O Christendom! For sinners, Jesus Christ became a companion of tax collectors and prostitutes: Rejoice, O Christendom! For the condemned, Jesus Christ was condemned to the cross on Golgotha: Rejoice, O Christendom! For all of us, Jesus Christ was resurrected to life: Rejoice, O Christendom! . . . All over the world today people are asking: Where is the path to joy? The church of Christ answers loudly: Jesus is our joy! (1 Pet. 1:7–9). Joy to the world!

Dietrich Bonhoeffer

In this you rejoice, even if now for a little while you have had to suffer various trials, so that the genuineness of your faith—being more precious than gold that, though perishable, is tested by fire—may be found to result in praise and glory and honor when Jesus Christ is revealed. Although you have not seen him, you love him; and even though you do not see him now, you believe in him and rejoice with an indescribable and glorious joy, for you are receiving the outcome of your faith, the salvation of your souls.

1 Peter 1:6–9

The Great Kingdom of Peace Has Begun

The authority of this poor child will grow (Isa. 9:7). It will encompass all the earth, and knowingly or unknowingly, all human generations until the end of the ages will have to serve it. It will be an authority over the hearts of people, but thrones and great kingdoms will also grow strong or fall apart with this power. The mysterious, invisible authority of the divine child over human hearts is more solidly grounded than the visible and resplendent power of earthly rulers. Ultimately all authority on earth must serve only the authority of Jesus Christ over humankind.

With the birth of Jesus, the great kingdom of peace has begun. Is it not a miracle that where Jesus has really become Lord over people, peace reigns? That there is one Christendom on the whole earth, in which there is peace in the midst of the world? Only where Jesus is not allowed to reign—where human stubbornness, defiance, hate, and avarice are allowed to live on unbroken—can there be no peace. Jesus does not want to set up his kingdom of peace by force, but where people willingly submit themselves to him and let him rule over them, he will give them his wonderful peace.

❖　❖　❖

I'm in the dark depths of night, and my thoughts are roaming far afield. Now that all the merry-making and rejoicing and candlelight are over and the noise and commotion of the day have been replaced by silence, inside and out, other voices can be heard. . . . The chill night wind and the mysterious darkness can open hearts and release forces that are unfathomable, but good and consoling. . . . Can you think of a better time than night-time? That's why Christ, too, chose to come to us—with his angels—at night.[1]

Maria von Wedemeyer to Bonhoeffer, December 25, 1943

❖ ❖ ❖

Now the birth of Jesus the Messiah took place in this way. When his mother Mary had been engaged to Joseph, but before they lived together, she was found to be with child from the Holy Spirit. Her husband Joseph, being a righteous man and unwilling to expose her to public disgrace, planned to dismiss her quietly. But just when he had resolved to do this, an angel of the Lord appeared to him in a dream and said, "Joseph, son of David, do not be afraid to take Mary as your wife, for the child conceived in her is from the Holy Spirit. She will bear a son, and you are to name him Jesus, for he will save his people from their sins." All this took place to fulfill what had been spoken by the Lord through the prophet:

"Look, the virgin shall conceive and bear a son,
    and they shall name him Emmanuel,"

which means, "God is with us." When Joseph awoke from sleep, he did as the angel of the Lord commanded him; he took her as his wife, but had no marital relations with her until she had borne a son; and he named him Jesus.

Matthew 1:18–25

On the Weak Shoulders of a Child

Authority rests upon his shoulders" (Isa. 9:6). Authority over the world is supposed to lie on the weak shoulders of this newborn child! One thing we know: these shoulders will come to carry the entire burden of the world. With the cross, all the sin and distress of this world will be loaded on these shoulders. But authority consists in the fact that the bearer does not collapse under the burden but carries it to the end. The authority that lies on the shoulders of the child in the manger consists in the patient bearing of people and their guilt. This bearing, however, begins in the manger; it begins where the eternal word of God assumes and bears human flesh. The authority over all the world has its beginning in the very lowliness and weakness of the child. . . . He accepts and carries the humble, the lowly, and sinners, but he rejects and brings to nothing the proud, the haughty, and the righteous (Luke 1:51–52).

From the Christian point of view there is no special problem about Christmas in a prison cell. For many people in this building it will probably be a more sincere and genuine occasion than in places where nothing but the name is kept. The misery, suffering, poverty, loneliness, helplessness, and guilt mean something quite different in the eyes of God from what they mean in the judgment of man, that

God will approach where men turn away, that Christ was born in a stable because there was no room for him in the inn—these are things that a prisoner can understand better than other people; for him they really are glad tidings.[2]

Bonhoeffer's letter to his parents from
Tegel prison, December 17, 1943

❖ ❖ ❖

Let the same mind be in you that was in Christ Jesus,
  who, though he was in the form of God,
    did not regard equality with God
    as something to be exploited,
  but emptied himself,
    taking the form of a slave,
    being born in human likeness.
  And being found in human form,
    he humbled himself
    and became obedient to the point of death—
    even death on a cross.

Therefore God also highly exalted him
    and gave him the name
    that is above every name,
  so that at the name of Jesus
    every knee should bend,
    in heaven and on earth and under the earth,
  and every tongue should confess
    that Jesus Christ is Lord,
    to the glory of God the Father.

Philippians 2:5–11

With God There Is Joy

Everlasting joy shall be upon their heads" (Isa. 35:10). Since ancient times, in the Christian church, acedia—sadness of heart, resignation—has been considered a mortal sin. "Serve the LORD with gladness!" (Ps. 100:2 RSV), urges the Scripture. For this, our life has been given to us, and for this, it has been sustained for us to this present hour. The joy that no one can take from us belongs not only to those who have been called home, but also to us who are still living. In this joy we are one with them, but never in sadness. How are we supposed to be able to help those who are without joy and courage, if we ourselves are not borne by courage and joy? What is meant here is not something made or forced, but something given and free. With God there is joy, and from him it comes down and seizes spirit, soul, and body. And where this joy has seized a person, it reaches out around itself, it pulls others along, it bursts through closed doors. There is a kind of joy that knows nothing at all of the pain, distress, and anxiety of the heart. But it cannot last; it can only numb for a time. The joy of God has gone through the poverty of the manger and the distress of the cross; therefore it is invincible and irrefutable.

❖　❖　❖

Acedia may be an unfamiliar term to those not well versed in monastic history or medieval literature. But that does not mean it has no relevance for contemporary readers. . . . I believe that such standard dictionary definitions of *acedia* as "apathy," "boredom," or "torpor" do not begin to cover it, and while we may find it convenient to regard it as a more primitive word for what we now term depression, the truth is much more complex. Having experienced both conditions, I think it likely that most of the restless boredom, frantic escapism, commitment phobia, and enervating despair that plagues us today is the ancient demon of acedia in modern dress.[3]

Kathleen Norris, *Acedia & Me: A Marriage,*
Monks, and a Writer's Life

❖　❖　❖

Make a joyful noise to the LORD, all the earth.
　Worship the LORD with gladness;
　come into his presence with singing.

Know that the LORD is God.
　It is he that made us, and we are his;
　we are his people, and the sheep of his pasture.

Enter his gates with thanksgiving,
　and his courts with praise.
　Give thanks to him, bless his name.

For the LORD is good;
　his steadfast love endures forever,
　and his faithfulness to all generations.

Psalm 100

Everlasting Father and Prince of Peace

Everlasting Father" (Isa. 9:6)—how can this be the name of the child? Only because in this child the everlasting fatherly love of God is revealed, and the child wants nothing other than to bring to earth the love of the Father. So the Son is one with the Father, and whoever sees the Son sees the Father. This child wants nothing for himself. He is no prodigy in the human sense, but an obedient child of his heavenly Father. Born in time, he brings eternity with him to earth; as Son of God he brings to us all the love of the Father in heaven. Go, seek, and find in the manger the heavenly Father who here has also become your dear Father.

"Prince of Peace"—where God comes in love to human beings and unites with them, there peace is made between God and humankind and among people. Are you afraid of God's wrath? Then go to the child in the manger and receive there the peace of God. Have you fallen into strife and hatred with your sister or brother? Come and see how God, out of pure love, has become our brother and wants to reconcile us with each other. In the world, power reigns. This child is the Prince of Peace. Where he is, peace reigns.

❖   ❖   ❖

In our lives we don't speak readily of victory. It is too big a word for us. We have suffered too many defeats in our lives; victory has been thwarted again and again by too many weak hours, too many gross sins. But isn't it true that the spirit within us yearns for this word, for the final victory over the sin and anxious fear of death in our lives? And now God's word also says nothing to us about our victory; it doesn't promise us that *we* will be victorious over sin and death from now own; rather, it says with all its might that someone has won this victory, and that this person, if we have him as Lord, will also win the victory over us. It is not we who are victorious, but Jesus.[4]

"Christus Victor" address, November 26, 1939

On that day, when evening had come, he said to them, "Let us go across to the other side." And leaving the crowd behind, they took him with them in the boat, just as he was. Other boats were with him. A great windstorm arose, and the waves beat into the boat, so that the boat was already being swamped. But he was in the stern, asleep on the cushion; and they woke him up and said to him, "Teacher, do you not care that we are perishing?" He woke up and rebuked the wind, and said to the sea, "Peace! Be still!" Then the wind ceased, and there was a dead calm. He said to them, "Why are you afraid? Have you still no faith?" And they were filled with great awe and said to one another, "Who then is this, that even the wind and the sea obey him?"

Mark 4:35–41

Beside Your Cradle Here I Stand

A verse is going around repeatedly in my head: "Brother, come; from all that grieves you / you are freed; / all you need / I again will bring you." What does this mean: "All you need I again will bring you"? Nothing is lost; in Christ everything is lifted up, preserved—to be sure, in a different form—transparent, clear, freed from the torment of self-seeking desire. Christ will bring all of this again, and as it was originally intended by God, without the distortion caused by our sin. The teaching of the gathering up of all things, found in Ephesians 1:10, is a wonderful and thoroughly comforting idea. "God seeks out what has gone by" (Eccl. 3:15) receives here its fulfillment. And no one has expressed that as simply and in such a childlike way as Paul Gerhardt in the words that he places in the mouth of the Christ child: "All you need I again will bring you." Moreover, for the first time in these days I have discovered for myself the song, "Beside your cradle here I stand." Until now I had not thought much about it. Apparently you have to be alone a long time and read it meditatively to be able to perceive it. . . . Beside the "we" there is also still an "I" and Christ, and what that means cannot be said better than in this song.

❖　❖　❖

When God's Son took on flesh, he truly and bodily took on, out of pure grace, our being, our nature, ourselves. This was the eternal counsel of the triune God. Now we are in him. Where he is, there we are too, in the incarnation, on the cross, and in his resurrection. We belong to him because we are in him. That is why the Scriptures call us the Body of Christ.[5]

Dietrich Bonhoeffer

With all wisdom and insight he has made known to us the mystery of his will, according to his good pleasure that he set forth in Christ, as a plan for the fullness of time, to gather up all things in him, things in heaven and things on earth. In Christ we have also obtained an inheritance, having been destined according to the purpose of him who accomplishes all things according to his counsel and will, so that we, who were the first to set our hope on Christ, might live for the praise of his glory.

Ephesians 1:8b–12

The Joyous Certainty of Faith

On the basis of God's beginning with us, which has already happened, our life with God is a path that is traveled in the law of God. Is this human enslavement under the law? No, it is liberation from the murderous law of incessant beginnings. Waiting day after day for the new beginning, thinking countless times that we have found it, only in the evening to give up on it again as lost—that is the perfect destruction of faith in the God who set the beginning once and for all time. . . . God has set the beginning: this is the joyous certainty of faith. Therefore, beside the "one" beginning of God, I am not supposed to try to set countless other beginnings of my own. This is precisely what I am now liberated from. The beginning—God's beginning—lies behind me, once and for all time. . . . Together we are on the path whose beginning consists in the fact that God has found his own people, a path whose end can consist only in the fact that God is seeking us again. The path between this beginning and this end is our walk in the law of God. It is life under the word of God in all its many facets. In truth there is only one danger on this path, namely, wanting to go behind the beginning. In that moment the path stops being a way of grace and faith. It stops being God's own way.

❖   ❖   ❖

I believe that God can and will bring good out of evil, even out of the greatest evil. For that purpose he needs men who make the best use of everything. I believe that God will give us all the strength we need to help us to resist in all times of distress. But he never gives it in advance, lest we should rely on ourselves and not on him alone. A faith such as this should allay all our fears for the future. I believe that even our mistakes and shortcomings are turned to good account, and that it is no harder for God to deal with them than with our supposedly good deeds. I believe that God is no timeless fate, but that he waits for and answers sincere prayers and responsible actions.[6]

"After Ten Years: A Reckoning Made
at New Year 1943"

We know that all things work together for good for those who love God, who are called according to his purpose. For those whom he foreknew he also predestined to be conformed to the image of his Son, in order that he might be the firstborn within a large family. And those whom he predestined he also called; and those whom he called he also justified; and those whom he justified he also glorified.

Romans 8:28–30

At the Beginning of a New Year

The road to hell is paved with good intentions." This saying, which is found in a broad variety of lands, does not arise from the brash worldly wisdom of an incorrigible. It instead reveals deep Christian insight. At the beginning of a new year, many people have nothing better to do than to make a list of bad deeds and resolve from now on—how many such "from-now-ons" have there already been!—to begin with better intentions, but they are still stuck in the middle of their paganism. They believe that a good intention already means a new beginning; they believe that on their own they can make a new start whenever they want. But that is an evil illusion: only God can make a new beginning with people whenever God pleases, but not people with God. Therefore, people cannot make a new beginning at all; they can only pray for one. Where people are on their own and live by their own devices, there is only the old, the past. Only where God is can there be a new beginning. We cannot command God to grant it; we can only pray to God for it. And we can pray only when we realize that we cannot do anything, that we have reached our limit, that someone else must make that new beginning.

❖　❖　❖

New Year's Text:

If we survive during the coming weeks or months, we shall be able to see quite clearly that all has turned out for the best. The idea that we could have avoided many of life's difficulties if we had taken things more cautiously is too foolish to be entertained for a moment. As I look back on your past I am so convinced that what has happened hitherto has been right, that I feel that what is happening now is right too. To renounce a full life and its real joys in order to avoid pain is neither Christian nor human.[7]

Bonhoeffer to Renate and Eberhard Bethge,
written from Tegel, January 23, 1944

❖ ❖ ❖

From now on, therefore, we regard no one from a human point of view; even though we once knew Christ from a human point of view, we know him no longer in that way. So if anyone is in Christ, there is a new creation: everything old has passed away; see, everything has become new!

2 Corinthians 5:16–17

Do Not Worry about Tomorrow

Possessions delude the human heart into believing that they provide security and a worry-free existence, but in truth they are the very cause of worry. For the heart that is fixed on possessions, they come with a suffocating burden of worry. Worries lead to treasure, and treasure leads back to worry. We want to secure our lives through possessions; through worry we want to become worry free, but the truth turns out to be the opposite. The shackles that bind us to possessions, that hold us fast to possessions, are themselves worries. The misuse of possessions consists in our using them for security for the next day. Worry is always directed toward tomorrow. In the strictest sense, however, possessions are intended only for today. It is precisely the securing of tomorrow that makes me so insecure today. "Today's trouble is enough for today" (Matt. 6:34b). Only those who place tomorrow in God's hands and receive what they need to live today are truly secure. Receiving daily liberates us from tomorrow. Thought for tomorrow delivers us up to endless worry.

❖ ❖ ❖

I have had the experience over and over again that the quieter it is around me, the clearer do I feel the connection to you. It is as though in solitude the soul develops senses which we hardly know in everyday life. Therefore I have not felt lonely or abandoned for one moment. You, the parents, all of you, the friends and students of mine at the front, all are constantly present to me. . . . Therefore you must not think me unhappy. What is happiness and unhappiness? It depends so little on the circumstances; it depends really only on that which happens inside a person.[8]

Bonhoeffer's final Christmastime letter to fiancée
Maria von Wedemeyer, December 19, 1944

❖   ❖   ❖

"Therefore do not worry, saying, 'What will we eat?' or 'What will we drink?' or 'What will we wear?' For it is the Gentiles who strive for all these things; and indeed your heavenly Father knows that you need all these things. But strive first for the kingdom of God and his righteousness, and all these things will be given to you as well.

"So do not worry about tomorrow, for tomorrow will bring worries of its own. Today's trouble is enough for today."

Matthew 6:31–34

A Necessary Daily Exercise

Why is it that my thoughts wander so quickly from God's word, and that in my hour of need the needed word is often not there? Do I forget to eat and drink and sleep? Then why do I forget God's word? Because I still can't say what the psalmist says: "I will delight in your statutes" (Ps. 119:16). I don't forget the things in which I take delight. Forgetting or not forgetting is a matter not of the mind but of the whole person, of the heart. I never forget what body and soul depend upon. The more I begin to love the commandments of God in creation and word, the more present they will be for me in every hour. Only love protects against forgetting.

Because God's word has spoken to us in history and thus in the past, the remembrance and repetition of what we have learned is a necessary daily exercise. Every day we must turn again to God's acts of salvation, so that we can again move forward. . . . Faith and obedience live on remembrance and repetition. Remembrance becomes the power of the present because of the living God who once acted for me and who reminds me of that today.

❖ ❖ ❖

In our meditation we ponder the chosen text on the strength of the promise that it has something utterly personal to say to us for this day and for our Christian life, that it is not only God's word for the Church, but also God's word for us individually. We expose ourselves to the specific word until it addresses us personally. And when we do this, we are doing no more than the simplest, untutored Christian does every day; we read God's word as God's word for us.[9]

Bonhoeffer, *Life Together*

❖   ❖   ❖

I treasure your word in my heart,
   so that I may not sin against you.
Blessed are you, O LORD;
   teach me your statutes.
With my lips I declare
   all the ordinances of your mouth.
I delight in the way of your decrees
   as much as in all riches.
I will meditate on your precepts,
   and fix my eyes on your ways.
I will delight in your statutes;
   I will not forget your word.

Deal bountifully with your servant,
   so that I may live and observe your word.
Open my eyes, so that I may behold
   wondrous things out of your law.

Psalm 119:11–18

For Everything There Is a Season

For those who find and give thanks to God in their earthly fortune, God will give them times in which to remember that all things on earth are only temporary, and that it is good to set one's heart on eternity. . . . All things have their time, and the main thing is to stay in step with God and not always be hurrying a few steps ahead or falling behind. To want everything all at once is to be overanxious. "For everything there is a season . . . to weep, and . . . to laugh; . . . to embrace, and . . . to refrain from embracing; . . . to tear, and . . . to sew . . ." (Eccl. 3:1a, 4a, 5b, 7a), "and God seeks out what has gone by" (3:15b). Yet this last part must mean that nothing past is lost, that with us God again seeks out the past that belongs to us. So when the longing for something past overtakes us—and this happens at completely unpredictable times—then we can know that this is only one of the many "times" that God makes available to us. And then we should not proceed on our own but seek out the past once again with God.

Dear Mother, I want you to know that I am constantly thinking of you and Father every day, and that I thank God for all that you are to me and the whole family. I know you've always lived for us and haven't lived a life of your own. . . . Thank you for all the love that has come to me in my cell from you during the past year, and has made every day easier for me. I think these hard years have brought us closer together than ever we were before. My wish for you and Father and Maria and for us all is that the New Year may bring us at least an occasional glimmer of light, and that we may once more have the opportunity of being together. May God keep you both well.[10]

Birthday letter to Bonhoeffer's mother
from prison, December 28, 1944

❖ ❖ ❖

For everything there is a season, and a time for every matter under heaven:
> a time to be born, and a time to die;
> a time to plant, and a time to pluck up what is
> > planted;
> a time to kill, and a time to heal;
> a time to break down, and a time to build up;
> a time to weep, and a time to laugh;
> a time to mourn, and a time to dance;
> a time to throw away stones, and a time to
> > gather stones together;
> a time to embrace, and a time to refrain from
> > embracing;
> a time to seek, and a time to lose;
> a time to keep, and a time to throw away;
> a time to tear, and a time to sew;
> a time to keep silence, and a time to speak;
> a time to love, and a time to hate;
> a time for war, and a time for peace.

Ecclesiastes 3:1–8

Morning by Morning He Wakens Me

Every new morning is a new beginning of our life. Every day is a completed whole. The present day should be the boundary of our care and striving (Matt. 6:34; Jas. 4:14). It is long enough for us to find God or lose God, to keep the faith or fall into sin and shame. God created day and night so that we might not wander boundlessly, but already in the morning may see the goal of the evening before us. As the old sun rises new every day, so the eternal mercies of God are new every morning (Lam. 3:22–23). To grasp the old faithfulness of God anew every morning, to be able—in the middle of life—to begin a new life with God daily, that is the gift that God gives with every new morning. . . .

Not fear of the day, not the burden of work that I have to do, but rather, the Lord wakens me. So says the servant of God: "Morning by morning he wakens—wakens my ear to listen as those who are taught" (Isa. 50:4c). God wants to open the heart before it opens itself to the world; before the ear hears the innumerable voices of the day, the early hours are the time to hear the voice of the Creator and Redeemer. God made the stillness of the early morning for himself. It ought to belong to God.

❖ ❖ ❖

Because intercession is such an incalculably great gift of God, we should accept it joyfully. The very time we give to intercession will turn out to be a daily source of new joy in God and in the Christian community. . . . For most people the early morning will prove to be the best time. We have a right to this time, even prior to the claims of other people, and we may insist upon having it as a completely undisturbed quiet time despite all external difficulties.[11]

Bonhoeffer, *Life Together*

The Lord GOD has given me
    the tongue of a teacher,
that I may know how to sustain
    the weary with a word.
Morning by morning he wakens —
    wakens my ear
        to listen as those who are taught.
Isaiah 50:4

The Feast of Epiphany

The curious uncertainty that surrounds the feast of Epiphany is as old as the feast itself. We know that long before Christmas was celebrated, Epiphany was the highest holiday in the Eastern and Western churches. Its origins are obscure, but it is certain that since ancient times this day has brought to mind four different events: the birth of Christ, the baptism of Christ, the wedding at Cana, and the arrival of the Magi from the East. . . . Be that as it may, since the fourth century the church has left the birth of Christ out of the feast of Epiphany. . . . The removal of the birth of Christ from his baptismal day had great significance. In gnostic and heretical circles in the East, the idea arose that the baptismal day was actually the day of Christ's birth as the Son of God. . . . But therein lay the possibility of a dangerous error, namely, a misunderstanding of God's incarnation. . . . If God had not accepted Jesus as his Son until Jesus' baptism, we would remain unredeemed. But if Jesus is the Son of God who from his conception and birth assumed our own flesh and blood, then and then alone is he true man and true God; only then can he help us; for then the "hour of salvation" for us has really come in his birth; then the birth of Christ is the salvation of all people.

❖ ❖ ❖

Today you will be baptized a Christian. All those great ancient words of the Christian proclamation will be spoken over you, and the command of Jesus Christ to baptize will be carried out on you, without your knowing anything about it. But we are once again being driven right back to the beginnings of our understanding. Reconciliation and redemption, regeneration and the Holy Spirit, love of our enemies, cross and resurrection, life in Christ and Christian discipleship.[12]

"Thoughts on the Baptism of
Dietrich Wilhelm Rüdiger Bethge,"
May 1944

When they had heard the king, they set out; and there, ahead of them, went the star that they had seen at its rising, until it stopped over the place where the child was. When they saw that the star had stopped, they were overwhelmed with joy. On entering the house, they saw the child with Mary his mother; and they knelt down and paid him homage. Then, opening their treasure chests, they offered him gifts of gold, frankincense, and myrrh. And having been warned in a dream not to return to Herod, they left for their own country by another road.

Matthew 2:9–12

NOTES

Editor's Preface

1. Stephen R. Haynes and Lori Brandt Hale, *Bonhoeffer for Armchair Theologians* (Louisville, Ky.: Westminster John Knox Press, 2009). See esp. 132–33 and 77–78.

2. Eberhard Bethge, *Dietrich Bonhoeffer: A Biography,* rev. ed. (Minneapolis: Fortress Press, 2000), 260.

3. Letter from Dietrich Bonhoeffer to Eberhard Bethge, November 21, 1943, in *Letters and Papers from Prison: New Greatly Enlarged Edition,* ed. Eberhard Bethge (New York: Touchstone, 1997), 135.

4. Haynes and Hale, *Bonhoeffer for Armchair Theologians,* 70–76.

Advent Week One: Waiting

1. Dietrich Bonhoeffer, *Dietrich Bonhoeffer's Christmas Sermons,* ed. and trans. Edwin Robertson (Grand Rapids: Zondervan, 2005), 171–72.

2. Ruth-Alice von Bismarck and Ulrich Kabitz, *Love Letters from Cell 92: The Correspondence between Dietrich Bonhoeffer and Maria von Wedemeyer, 1943–45* (Nashville: Abingdon Press, 1992), 133.

3. *Ibid.,* 128.

4. Dietrich Bonhoeffer, "The Coming of Jesus in Our Midst," in *Watch for the Light: Readings for Advent and Christmas* (Maryknoll, N.Y.: Orbis Books, 2001), 205.

5. Dietrich Bonhoeffer, *I Want to Live These Days with You* (Louisville, Ky.: Westminster John Knox Press, 2007), 369.

6. Bonhoeffer, *Letters and Papers from Prison*, 135.

7. Bonhoeffer, *I Want to Live These Days with You*, 366.

Advent Week Two: Mystery

1. Bonhoeffer, *I Want to Live These Days with You*, 152.

2. Bismarck and Kabitz, *Love Letters from Cell 92*, 138.

3. Bonhoeffer, *I Want to Live These Days with You*, 149.

4. Brennan Manning, *The Ragamuffin Gospel Visual Edition* (Sisters, Ore.: Multnomah Publishers, 2005), n.p.

5. Bonhoeffer, *I Want to Live These Days with You*, 377.

6. Eugene Peterson, "Introduction," in *God with Us: Rediscovering the Meaning of Christmas*, ed. Greg Pennoyer and Gregory Wolfe (Brewster, Mass.: Paraclete Press, 2007), 1.

7. Scott Cairns, in *God with Us*, 57.

Advent Week Three: Redemption

1. Dietrich Bonhoeffer, *A Testament to Freedom: The Essential Writings of Dietrich Bonhoeffer*, ed. Geffrey B. Kelly and F. Burton Nelson (San Francisco: HarperOne, 1990, 1995), 217.

2. Bonhoeffer, *Dietrich Bonhoeffer's Christmas Sermons*, 22–23.

3. Ibid., 103–4.

4. Bonhoeffer, *Testament to Freedom*, 223.

5. Bonhoeffer, *Letters and Papers from Prison*, 323.

6. Bonhoeffer, *Testament to Freedom*, 185–86.

7. Ibid., 218.

Advent Week Four: Incarnation

1. Bonhoeffer, *Dietrich Bonhoeffer's Christmas Sermons*, 151. By Christmas of 1940, the Nazis had forbidden Bonhoeffer to preach publicly. This excerpt comes from a Christmas sermon he wrote that was circulated in print.

2. Frederica Mathewes-Green, *At the Corner of East and Now: A Modern Life in Ancient Christian Orthodoxy* (New York: Penguin Putnam, 1999), posted online at http://www.frederica.com/east-now-excerpt-1/.

3. Bonhoeffer, *Dietrich Bonhoeffer's Christmas Sermons*, 38–39.

4. Ibid., 151–52.

5. Ibid., 37.

6. Luci Shaw, in *God with Us*, 77–78.

7. Bismarck and Kabitz, *Love Letters from Cell 92*, 132.

The Twelve Days of Christmas

1. Bismarck and Kabitz, *Love Letters from Cell 92*, 145.

2. Bonhoeffer, *Letters and Papers from Prison*, 166.

3. Kathleen Norris, *Acedia & Me: A Marriage, Monks, and a Writer's Life* (New York: Riverhead, 2008), 2–3.

4. In *Dietrich Bonhoeffer: Writings Selected with an Introduction by Robert Coles* (Maryknoll, N.Y.: Orbis Books, 1998), 88.

5. Dietrich Bonhoeffer, *Life Together: The Classic Exploration of Christian Community* (New York: Harper, 1954), 24.

6. In *Dietrich Bonhoeffer: Writings*, 111–12. This New Year's reflection was written by Bonhoeffer in 1943 and circulated in a small way among his friends and coconspirators against Hitler, but it was not published until after his death.

7. Bonhoeffer, *Letters and Papers from Prison*, 191.

8. Ibid., 419.

9. Bonhoeffer, *Life Together*, 82.

10. In *Dietrich Bonhoeffer: Writings*, 126–27.

11. Bonhoeffer, *Life Together*, 87.

12. Bonhoeffer, *Testament to Freedom*, 504–5.

SCRIPTURE INDEX

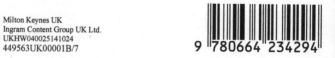

9 780664 234294

God Is in
the Manger

DIETRICH BONHOEFFER

God Is in the Manger

Reflections on Advent and Christmas

TRANSLATED BY O. C. DEAN JR.

COMPILED AND EDITED BY JANA RIESS

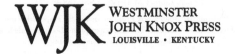

♾ The paper used in this publication meets the minimum requirements of the
American National Standard for Information Sciences—Permanence of Paper for
Printed Library Materials, ANSI Z39.48-1992.

Westminster John Knox Press advocates the responsible use
of our natural resources. The text paper of this book is made from
at least 30% post-consumer waste.

THE GREAT PHYSICIAN'S

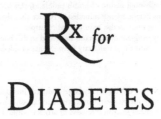

DIABETES

JORDAN RUBIN

with Joseph Brasco, M.D.

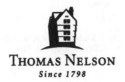

THOMAS NELSON
Since 1798

NASHVILLE   DALLAS   MEXICO CITY   RIO DE JANEIRO   BEIJING

© 2006 by Jordan Rubin

Published in Nashville, Tennessee, by Thomas Nelson. Thomas Nelson is a trademark of Thomas Nelson, Inc.

Thomas Nelson, Inc. titles may be purchased in bulk for educational, business, fund-raising, or sales promotional use. For information, please e-mail SpecialMarkets@ThomasNelson.com.

Scripture quotations are from the NEW KING JAMES VERSION®. © 1979, 1980, 1982 by Thomas Nelson, Inc. Used by permission. All rights reserved.

Library of Congress Cataloging-in-Publication Data

Rubin, Jordan.
    The Great Physician's Rx for diabetes / by Jordan Rubin with Joseph Brasco.
        p. cm.
    Includes bibliographical references (p.   ).
        ISBN: 0785297480

    1. Diabetes—Popular works. 2. Diabetes—Religious aspects—Christianity. 3. Diabetics—Rehabilitation—Popular works. I. Brasco, Joseph. II. Title.
RC660.4.R84 2006
616.4'6206—dc22   2005036830

Printed in the United States of America

08 09 10 11 QW 15 14 13

To my Great Grandpa Jacob and Great Grandma Leah, who suffered terribly and died from complications related to diabetes, and to the millions today who endure this painful condition. May this book offer you hope.

CONTENTS

CONTENTS

INTRODUCTION

Time to Make a Change

I n early 2004, Joey Hinson sat attentively while I spoke at a Wednesday night service at my home church, Christ Fellowship Church, in Palm Beach Gardens, Florida. That evening, I described how a thirty-nine-year-old acquaintance of mine had suddenly died from a heart attack, leaving behind a beautiful wife, four energetic kids, and a thriving ministry. "I had been asked to speak to this father and husband about getting on God's health plan, but we never connected in time," I said that evening. "How would his life—and those who mattered most to him—have changed if he had managed to turn around his health in time?"

A year later my church asked me to speak again, and this time Joey introduced himself after the service. "When you spoke a year ago, that story about that thirty-nine-year-old guy really did a number on me. You see, I'm also a husband and a father, and I felt like you were speaking directly to me. I knew I had to do something."

"Tell me about it," I said, intrigued, but humbled by what I had heard.

After he finished describing the events of the past year, I asked Joey if we could share his story with readers of *The Great Physician's Rx for Diabetes*. Here's what happened, in his words:

Throughout much of 2003, I began feeling horrible. This was something new for me because I thought I was in good shape, even for a guy who had turned fifty. I had played football in college—I lined up as an offensive lineman at Mars Hill College in North Carolina—so I was encouraged to "eat big" when I was growing up. It was hard to get away from that mentality after my college days were over, however. Over the years, I gained some weight—probably a good twenty or thirty pounds extra on my six-foot, two-inch frame. When I tipped the scales at 250 pounds a few years ago, I told myself to do something about it. I attended so many Weight Watchers meetings that I received a lifetime membership, but once I went off their food, the weight always came right back.

I think it's because I liked to eat southern foods too much. My weakness was fried chicken, black-eyed peas, and collard greens with the ham bone cooked in, or country-fried steaks dripping with gravy and yellow rice. Dessert had to be a rich chocolate cake or pecan pie.

Cheeseburgers and fries worked just fine for lunch. I worked as the transportation director at King's Academy, a private Christian school near my hometown of Royal Palm Beach, Florida, and a couple of times a week I borrowed the school's golf cart and drove to the Wendy's or Burger King located next door to school. People looked at me funny when they saw me ordering lunch from my golf cart, but I didn't mind. I was having fun.

What wasn't fun was experiencing a shortness of breath and lack of energy after turning fifty. Our house has a good-sized lawn that usually takes me several hours to mow. In the muggy Florida summer heat, I was too pooped to tackle the project. I'd lie down on the sofa, gasping for air, frightened by how fast my heart was beating. I felt really bad.

Donna, my wife, was naturally concerned, and I was bothered that I didn't have the energy to keep up with our youngest son, a ten-year-old. Then one Sunday night in August 2003, I was sitting in church, listening to the pastor, when beads of sweat formed on my forehead. My heart thumped like a bass drum, and I feared that a heart attack was imminent. "Lord, what should I do?" I prayed. Things got so scary that I thought about signaling for an usher to call 911, but I didn't want to create a scene in the middle of a church service.

I thought I was having high blood pressure problems since hypertension ran in the family. My symptoms calmed down a bit, so I toughed it out. I knew I should see a doctor, but I decided to wait a week or two for my annual physical. After my doctor poked and prodded around, he ordered tests on my blood and urine.

I'll never forget the phone call from the doctor's office informing me that I had type 2 diabetes.

Diabetes? That sounded serious. "Wait a minute," I said to the nurse. "I had my physical in the afternoon, so

I'm not sure if I fasted for my blood work. I want to get this checked again."

A repeat visit confirmed the test results. "I'm going to write you a prescription," my doctor said, handing me a slip and sending me on my way.

My prescription was for thirty milligrams of Actos daily to treat type 2 diabetes. As the months passed, however, I can't say that I was feeling better or that the medication helped me regain my energy. My concerns were raised by newspaper stories that Actos could cause liver damage.

Then I heard Jordan Rubin speak about the Great Physician's prescription for good health, and his message inspired me to make huge lifestyle changes in what I ate and how I lived. I asked Donna if we could buy our groceries at the health food store and purchase some of the whole food nutritional supplements that Jordan recommended. I think she fell over in shock because she had been encouraging me for years to live a healthier lifestyle.

I began eating a healthy diet filled with fruits, vegetables, and the right type of dairy, eggs, and meats. The days of ordering food at the Wendy's drive-thru lane in a golf cart were long gone. Energy returned to the point that I could mow my big lawn again and keep up with the kids. Within a year, I had lost forty pounds and got down to my old high school playing weight.

When my annual physical came around in August 2004, I visited a new physician, but I did not disclose that I had been told a year earlier that I had diabetes. I wanted him to treat me with no preconceptions. So you can imagine my surprise when the test results from the lab confirmed that my cholesterol was good, my blood pressure was normal, and everything else was fine, meaning I didn't have diabetes.

Wow! Jordan Rubin was right. He said that if I followed the Great Physician's prescription, there would be a good chance that I'd reverse the damage I'd done to my body, and that's exactly what happened.

THE LATEST EPIDEMIC

Meeting people like Joey Hinson and hearing their stories are awesome, but my ears always perk up when someone says he has diabetes. You see, I had my own battle with diabetes back when I was a nineteen-year-old student at Florida State University a little more than a decade ago.

I chronicled my health odyssey in *The Great Physician's Rx for Health and Wellness*, where I described how my 185-pound body was attacked by Crohn's disease—a debilitating digestive order—along with a grab bag of other ailments: arthritis, chronic fatigue, hair loss, amebic dysentery, chronic candidiasis, prostate and bladder infections, as well as diabetes. Within a year I wasted away to 104 pounds and feared an early death.

Because I was fighting battles on so many medical fronts, I wasn't your typical diabetes patient, but I've never forgotten how both of my lower legs turned purple from extremely poor circulation. Now *that* got my attention. Although my doctors never suggested that I was a candidate for amputation, the thought of losing a leg crossed my young mind. If my health degenerated to a point where amputation was necessary, I really thought I would be better off dying.

Fortunately, and with great gratitude to my Lord and Savior, my health gradually improved, and the circulation in my legs returned to normal. Ever since I got well, I've carried a healthy respect for how diabetes impacts people's lives, and that impact is expected to double worldwide in the next twenty-five years. Researchers at the University of Edinburgh in Scotland are projecting a global rise in diabetes from 171 million in 2000 to 366 million in 2030. The greatest relative increases will occur in the Middle Eastern crescent, sub-Saharan Africa, and India, matching a similar rise in obesity rates.

Here in the United States, the alarm has already been sounded regarding diabetes. According to the most recent government statistics, around 18 million Americans—or 6.3 percent of the population—have been diagnosed with diabetes, and researchers estimate that there may be almost as many undiagnosed diabetics. The disease displays a strong ethnic bias based on its prevalence, in terms of percentage, among Native Americans, African-Americans, and Hispanics, as well as the aged.

Diabetes kills more than 200,000 Americans every year, ranking it as the sixth leading cause of death. Health authorities, however, believe that diabetes is underreported as a cause of death because many families and doctors, for one reason or another, choose not to enter the disease on the death certificate. A probable reason is that people often die of complications *relating* to diabetes—heart disease, strokes, high blood pressure, and kidney disease—so that disease becomes recorded as the cause of death.

Thus, many people are unaware that they even have diabetes. Although the affliction trails cancer and heart disease by considerable margins in the cause-of-death department, medical practitioners are calling diabetes a runaway epidemic because an estimated 41 million Americans have pre-diabetes, according to government estimates. Pre-diabetes is the period when people at high risk for developing full-blown diabetes demonstrate signs of intermittent elevated blood sugar levels. While their bodies are still capable of processing glucose—the energy that fuels the body's cells—their blood sugar levels are spiking like an aggressive teen driver running up the RPMs on his tachometer.

The "redline" image is apropos, especially since the American Diabetes Association has come out with red plastic wristbands as a way of creating awareness for the disease, just as cyclist Lance Armstrong introduced the canary yellow "Live Strong" wristbands as a fund-raiser for cancer research.

BACKGROUND ON DIABETES

Although millions of Americans and their families are affected by diabetes, I would venture to say that most people have a vague awareness of what diabetes entails. By definition, diabetes is a chronic degenerative disease caused by the body's inability to either produce enough insulin or properly use insulin, which is essential for the proper metabolism of blood sugar, also known as glucose. For those of you who last heard about insulin back in high school biology class, insulin is a hormone the body uses to convert sugar, starches, and other foods into energy for the cells.

To help you better understand the role of insulin, let me offer a short and simple description of how the body digests and absorbs food. The body's digestive process is considerably more complex than the following word picture, but this will give a general idea of how insulin is injected into the bloodstream.

When someone eats a meal, food travels from the mouth into the stomach before passing into the small intestines, much like the way food moves along various conveyor belts on *Unwrapped,* the Food Network program that shows viewers how their favorite foods are manufactured. Just as the featured item on *Unwrapped* is glazed, salted, roasted, or sugared as it wends its way through the factory, the food in the digestive tract is sprayed with various hormones, chemicals, and digestive juices. When food reaches the small intestines, it's bombarded with pancreatic juice containing pancreatic or digestive enzymes, which breaks the carbohydrates in the food down to the simplest form, glucose, which converts to blood sugar. When blood sugar levels rise, insulin is released to lower the blood sugar levels back to the normal range. The more carbohydrates you eat that are converted into blood sugar, the more your body releases insulin to lower that blood sugar.

Insulin accomplishes several tasks worth mentioning. The introduction of insulin stimulates the body to make fats out of other nutrients—proteins and especially carbohydrates—through a process known as lipogenesis. Why does the body do this? Because your body never wants to be caught short of gas in the tank. By storing the energy contained in sugar—or glucose—in fat cells, the body can call upon these "reserves" following physical exertion.

Unfortunately, with the lack of exercise in our couch-potato world these days, those reserves rarely get called on. Result: insulin levels spring out of whack after fat cells hang around too long. When blood sugar levels yo-yo for a long enough time, *diabetes mellitus* rears its ugly head in two forms: type 1 or type 2 diabetes. Doctors, however, are seeing increasing numbers of patients with double diabetes—symptoms of type 1 and type 2 diabetes.

Type 1, known as an insulin-dependent diabetes, means that the body does not produce enough insulin. To make up for the insulin deficit, the body must be supplied with steady amounts of insulin through a combination of controlled diet and daily injections of insulin, either extracted from the pancreases of cows or pigs or produced in laboratories in a synthetic form. In the last thirty years, medical scientists have discovered a way of manufacturing human insulin in bacteria and yeast, thanks to advancements in recombinant-DNA technology. Diabetics do not have to rely on insulin harvested from cows or pigs, whose supplies are being pinched by the limited number of animals set aside for this purpose.

Injections must be delivered with a needle because swallowing insulin is ineffective, the reason being that digestive juices in the mouth destroy insulin (which is a protein) before it reaches the bloodstream. My heart goes out to type 1 diabetics since it has to be incredibly painful and inconvenient to inject yourself in the thigh, arm, or abdomen every single day of your life. A new treatment protocol involves the use of an insulin pump, a small computerized device that delivers insulin into the body through a thin tube and needle inserted in the skin, usually somewhere around the beltline. I know several type 1 diabetics who are extremely thankful that their doctors switched them from injections to the pump, claiming that action has saved their lives.

Type 2 diabetes, a form of *non*-insulin-dependent diabetes (although some type 2 diabetics get so bad that they often require insulin), is difficult to diagnose and more challenging to treat. With type 2 diabetes, the pancreas does not produce enough insulin, or the cells ignore the insulin produced by the body. Since insulin regulates and maintains the body's circulation of sugar levels, the body's inability to metabolize blood sugar—for whatever reason—opens the door to a host of medical complications.

Insulin resistance by the body's cells may be caused by too much insulin production—a by-product of a high-sugar, high-starch diet. Insulin resistance can be compared to building up a callus while working a hoe in the backyard: when too much insulin is produced, the cells build up a defense, causing large amounts of sugar to remain in the blood. Often, the sugar in the blood reacts with the proteins to form advanced glycation end products, which hinder blood flow to the eyes, legs, and feet. Eating foods with antioxidants can stop their formation.

In addition to poor blood circulation, some of the common symptoms of type 2 diabetes include increased thirst, frequent urination, dry, itchy skin, poor wound healing, fatigue, bad breath, and irritability. The symptoms may sound vague, but in combination, these give a clearer indication of the onset of the disease. When full-blown diabetes is diagnosed—and the disease begins to take hold—additional physical problems and side effects become more stark: kidney failure, eye problems possibly leading to blindness, tooth and gum infections, and circulation blockages that cause heart disease or heart attacks. Some diabetic patients discover they have neurological problems and poor circulation, which manifest as tingly feelings in the hands or feet.

Diabetes is a leading cause of blindness, kidney failure, limb amputations, and heart disease. There's also a huge link between the rising rates of obesity in this country and the "epidemic" of type 2 diabetes. The fact that our government classifies two-thirds of Americans as overweight and 15 percent of children between the ages of six and nineteen as severely overweight does not bode well for the future of this country.

This is how serious type 2 diabetes is among the young: some demographers are worried that today's generation could be the first to live fewer years than today's life expectancy, which is 72.5 years for men and 78.9 years for women, according to the National Center for Health Statistics. Furthermore, researchers say that if present trends continue, one out of three children born after 2000 will develop type 2 diabetes, and those who develop type 2 diabetes before the age of fifteen will have a shortened life expectancy of approximately fifteen years.[1] That's sobering news, especially to someone who became a father for the first time in 2004.

CONVENTIONAL TREATMENTS

Diabetes is a serious disease that has no cure. The disease can be somewhat controlled, however, but that involves lifelong treatment and attention. Type 1 diabetics take daily insulin shots to maintain their blood sugar level within a normal or near normal range. Type 2 diabetics manage the disease through diet, exercise, and medication under the supervision of a physician.

Type 1 diabetics must monitor their blood sugar levels several times a day, incorporate thirty minutes of exercise into their daily activities, and spread their intake of carbohydrates throughout the day to prevent high blood sugar levels after meals. Insulin is the only medication used to treat diabetes directly, although some doctors prescribe medications like Cymbalta to treat depression or painful nerve damage in the hands or feet.

Type 2 medical treatments are more individualized. Doctors will focus on treatment plans that stabilize blood sugar levels, which revolve around eating the proper amount of carbohydrates each day. Since carbohydrates are the nutrients that most affect blood sugar, doctors will counsel their patients to "count carbs" so that they can maintain their blood sugar at a safe level. Registered dietitians are usually brought in to teach patients how to plan meals and count carbohydrates. Unfortunately, the current standard medical and dietetic recommendations are that diabetics substitute sugar and sugar-containing foods with artificial sweeteners and artificially sweetened products.

Doctors often recommend a low-fat, low-sodium diet with foods high in fiber to help balance blood sugar levels. Depending on their diagnosis, they may prescribe drugs that stimulate the pancreas to produce more insulin. Sulfa-containing compounds such as Glucotrol, DiaBeta, Micronase, or Prandin squeeze more insulin out of the body's cells. Other drugs help the body become more insulin sensitive: Avandamet, Rosiglitazone, and Metformin.

WHERE WE GO FROM HERE

From here on out, when I talk about diabetes, I will be referring to type 2 diabetes. My main reason is that more than 90 percent of diabetics are type 2, and the rapid increase in this form of the disease is prompting the alerts of an epidemic on the horizon. In addition, type 1 diabetes is thought to be largely an immune system disorder, and some in the medical world believe it's an autoimmune disease caused by a latent virus. More important, there is no proven way to prevent type 1 diabetes, but considerable evidence suggests that type 2 diabetes is highly preventable through eating right, living an overall healthy lifestyle, and embarking on an exercise program.

I believe even more can be done to prevent type 2 diabetes, and in the next seven chapters, I will be sharing the Great Physician's seven keys to health and wellness, which will give you and your loved ones the best possible chance to prevent diabetes or help you overcome diabetes by augmenting the medical treatment you're receiving.

My approach to diabetes is based on seven keys established in my foundational book, *The Great Physician's Rx for Health and Wellness:*

- Key #1: Eat to live.

- Key #2: Supplement your diet with whole food nutritionals, living nutrients, and superfoods.

- Key #3: Practice advanced hygiene.

- Key #4: Condition your body with exercise and body therapies.

- Key #5: Reduce toxins in your environment.

- Key #6: Avoid deadly emotions.

- Key #7: Live a life of prayer and purpose.

Each of these keys relates in some way to diabetes, as you will see. I believe each and every one of us has a God-given health potential that can be unlocked only with the right keys. I'm asking you to give the Bible's health plan a chance and incorporate these timeless principles into your life, allowing God to transform your health physically, mentally, emotionally, and spiritually.

No matter where you are in your health journey, I pray that God will meet you at your deepest point of need and deliver you from your health challenges.

Key # 1

Eat to Live

If you or a loved one has type 2 diabetes, you've probably noticed that friends and acquaintances who *don't* have this disease are often confused about your medical condition. They figure diabetes has something to do with sugar, but that's often the extent of their knowledge.

The general public harbors many misconceptions about diabetes. Some believe you're a prime candidate to develop diabetes if you're a closet chocoholic. This isn't exactly true; excessive consumption of sweets is more likely to give you a mouthful of cavities than cause diabetes. The body's inability to produce the right amount of insulin is the problem, not a secret love affair with Swiss chocolate. While everyone in the medical community agrees that sweets do raise blood glucose levels, people with diabetes can safely eat sugar. Diabetics shouldn't eat too much sugar, as I'll explain later in this chapter.

Others believe that diabetes can't be prevented. They say there's a strong hereditary link for those with a family history of diabetes, and if your parents have diabetes, then that's your destiny as well. While diabetes exhibits a strong hereditary component, "its rate of increase is too great to be a consequence of increased gene frequency," wrote Lyle MacWilliam in *LifeExtension* magazine. "Instead, evidence points toward the combined influences of lifestyle, dietary, and environmental factors."[1]

A generation ago, type 2 diabetes was unheard of among children, but the escalating numbers of youngsters with diabetes assert that the incidence of this childhood disease will become very serious over the next few decades. Experts are noting that type 2 diabetes is showing up with alarming regularity in heavy-set children who lead sedentary lives.

That's why I believe there's a link—medically and statistically—between the swelling ranks of diabetics and the other epidemic on everyone's lips—obesity. Not all overweight adults or children have diabetes, but it appears that nearly all type 2 diabetics are overweight. You need to look no further than a doctor's examination room for confirmation. Doctors on the front lines say that 99 percent of their patients with type 2 diabetes fit the preferred medical definition of overweight or obese, which is a body mass index (BMI) of 25 or 30 or more, respectively.

The body mass index is a mathematical formula that takes into account a person's height and weight and comes up with a corresponding number called the BMI. As a strict formula, the body mass index equals a person's weight in kilograms divided in height by meters squared. According to a body mass index table converted to pounds and inches for American use (these indexes are easily available online), the BMI breakdown goes like this:

- 18 or lower: underweight
- 19–24: normal
- 25–29: overweight
- 30–39: obese
- 40–54: extremely obese

As an example, someone standing five feet ten inches tall and weighing 167 pounds would have a BMI of 24—the limit defining one as having normal weight. Someone with the same height and weighing more than 209 pounds would have a BMI of 30, earning him or her a classification of obese on the body mass index scale. (Those who lift weights and have a large amount of lean body mass will be considered overweight or obese, according to the BMI scale. If you have a high BMI with a low percentage of body fat, you are not overweight or obese. This scale was created for the average nonathletic individual.)

If you find yourself on the upper end of the BMI scale, this would be an excellent time to ask your doctor about whether you should submit to diabetes testing, which usually involves a fasting blood glucose test or an oral glucose tolerance test. When the results come back from the lab, your doctor will inform you whether you have normal blood glucose, prediabetes, or diabetes. If the news is the latter, you will probably be counseled to lose some weight, undertake a regular exercise program, and reduce stress in your life—all ingredients of a major lifestyle change.

Losing weight is a *great* way to reduce the stranglehold that diabetes has on your body. A U.S. federally funded study called the Diabetes Prevention Program showed that losing between 5 percent and 7 percent of your body weight significantly reduces the risk of type 2 diabetes because a body carrying less weight uses insulin more effectively.

The Great Physician's Rx for Diabetes relies heavily on my first key, "Eat to live," which is an effective tool for losing weight. How does one eat to live? By doing two things:

1. Eat what God created for food.

2. Eat food in a form that is healthy for the body.

These principles involve eating foods and drinking liquids that give you an excellent chance of shedding pounds and maintaining the correct blood sugar levels. It doesn't mean exiting doughnut shops, fast-food restaurants, and supermarket checkout lines carrying bags of processed foods pumped up with sugars and artificial ingredients. Eating foods that God created in a form healthy for the body means choosing foods that allow you to beat back diseases like diabetes and put you on the road toward living a healthy, vibrant life.

For those with diabetes, this means consuming generous amounts of quality proteins, eating less high-glycemic carbohydrates such as grains, sugars, breads, pastas, rice, potatoes, and corn, and consuming more low-glycemic carbohydrates such as most vegetables and fruits, nuts, seeds, and legumes, and small amounts of whole grains.

When it comes to eating (1) foods that God created (2) in a form healthy for the body, I'm convinced that a diet based on consuming whole and natural foods fits within the bull's-eye of eating to live. Yet too many of the so-called foods sold in our nation's supermarkets were not created by God but were produced by employees in hairnets on an assembly line at some far-flung factory.

Like sheep following the next one off a cliff, we are filling our shopping carts with processed foods missing many of the nutrients that God intended us to receive and fortified with "modern" additives that rob us of health and vitality. As for eating out, don't get me started on how we've become a country that loves deep-fried, greasy food high in calories, high in fat, high in sugar, and—in most people's minds—high in taste.

Eating foods that God created in a form healthy for the body is an instant way to consume fewer calories. According to the Mayo Clinic, you consume only sixty calories when you eat one of these foods as a snack:

- one small apple
- one-half cup of grapes
- two plums
- two tablespoons of raisins
- one and one-half cups of strawberries
- two cups of shredded lettuces
- one-half cup of diced tomatoes
- two cups of spinach
- three-fourths cup of green beans

On the other hand, a Burger King Double Whopper with cheese comes out to a whopping 1,150 calories, or *twice* the amount of calories contained in *all* the fruits and vegetables I just listed!

I will be the first to agree that a diet of fruits and vegetables is too simplistic—and boring. Besides, a diet of low-cal fruits and vegetables does not provide the body with the full slate of nutrients that it needs, such as healthy proteins and fats. But let's get real: too many Americans are exiting fast-food restaurants, ice cream emporiums, and supermarket checkout lines with processed foods pumped up with calories like weight lifters on steroids. That's why we're having a nationwide problem with diabetes and obesity.

Contrary to popular opinion, there is no "diabetes diet." Foods healthy for everyone are foods that control blood glucose levels, but you must consume your foods carefully, especially carbohydrates. Every bite you take, whether it's a protein, fat, or carbohydrate, impacts your blood sugar and metabolism—and therefore your diabetes. Let's take a closer look at these macronutrients.

PROTEINS ARE PRACTICALLY PERFECT

Proteins, one of the basic components of nutrition, are the essential building blocks of the body. All proteins are combinations of twenty-two amino acids, which build body organs, muscles, and nerves, to name a few important duties. Among other things, proteins provide for the transport of nutrients, oxygen, and waste throughout the body and are required for the structure, function, and regulation of the body's cells, tissues, and organs.

Our bodies, however, cannot produce all twenty-two amino acids that we need to live a robust life. Scientists have discovered that eight essential amino acids are missing, meaning that they must come from other sources outside the body.

Since we need those eight amino acids badly, it just so happens that animal protein—chicken, beef, lamb, dairy, and eggs—is the only complete protein source providing the Big Eight amino acids.

The body needs the amino acids found in animal proteins, and the best and most healthy sources are organically raised cattle, sheep, goats, buffalo, and venison. Grass-fed meat is leaner and lower in calories than grain-fed beef. Organic and grass-fed beef is higher in heart-friendly omega-3 fatty acids and important vitamins like B$_{12}$ and E, and is way better for you than assembly-line cuts of flank steak from hormone-injected cattle eating pesticide-sprayed feed laced with antibiotics. Eating protein supports weight loss and healthy blood sugar levels.

Fish with fins and scales caught from oceans and rivers are lean sources of protein and provide essential amino acids in abundance. Supermarkets are stocking these types of foods in greater quantities these days, and of course, they are found in natural food stores, fish markets, and specialty stores.

FAT OBSESSION

When I was a college student in the mid-1990s, I can remember sitting in the Florida State cafeteria and watching the coeds pick through their lunchtime salads while obsessing about the number of fat grams in the dressing. Low-fat diets were the craze back then, and anything with fat in it was Public Enemy No. 1. The thinking went along these lines, especially for the girls: *If you eat something with fat, then it will make you fat.*

As it turned out, consuming low-fat, reduced-fat, or fat-free foods didn't help anyone lose weight and may have actually caused metabolic problems. The problem with reduced-fat chips and fat-free yogurt was more than their poor taste: it turned out that these convenience foods had nearly the same amount of calories as the "full fat" versions. Since people thought they were eating low-fat, healthy food, they ate with abandon, which caused many to gain weight.

There's a compelling reason why low-fat foods were not the hoped for panacea. Chemically altered foods make things worse for the body, not better. God, in His infinite wisdom, created fats as a concentrated source of energy and source material for cell membranes and various hormones. Fats give foods flavor and aroma by adding creaminess, shine, smoothness, and moisture. In addition, fats are responsible for regenerating healthy tissues and maintaining ideal body composition, and they carry the fat-soluble vitamins A, D, E, and K throughout the body.

What types of fats in foods should diabetics eat? Ron Rosedale, M.D., author of *The Rosedale Diet* (Collins, 2004), believes that nuts, seeds, and nut and seed butters are great sources of fats that help buffer insulin (less insulin helps insulin sensitivity) and trigger the brain that the body is full.

People are often shocked to hear me say this, but this is why I say butter is better for you than margarine. Organically produced butter is loaded with healthy fats such as short-chain saturated fatty acids, which supply energy to the body and aid in the regeneration of the digestive tract. Margarine, on the other hand, is a man-made, congealed conglomeration of chemicals and hydrogenated liquid vegetable oils.

Fats and oils created by God, as you would expect, are fats you want to include in your diet. The top two on my list are extra virgin coconut and olive oils, which are beneficial to the body and aid metabolism. I urge you to cook with extra virgin coconut oil, which is a near miracle food that few people have ever heard of.

A SPOONFUL OF SUGAR

Of the different macronutrients—proteins, fats, and carbohydrates—carbohydrates have the biggest effect on blood sugar levels. Eating too many carbohydrates—especially those from refined sources—is a forerunner for diabetes because the body has a limited capacity to store excess carbohydrates. Too many carbs force the body to convert the excess carbohydrates into stored body fat.

By definition, carbohydrates are the sugars and starches contained in plant foods. Sugars and starches, like fats, are not bad for you, but the problem for those fighting diabetes is that the standard American diet includes way too many foods containing these carbohydrates. People with diabetes are usually careful about their intake of sugar, but you should be aware that sugar does not raise blood sugar levels any differently than similar amounts of calories from the starches found in many foods.

Still, health-care providers rightfully recommend that you avoid eating sugar unnecessarily, but that is easier said than done. Sugar and its sweet relatives—high fructose corn syrup, sucrose, molasses, and maple syrup—are among the first ingredients listed in staples such as cereals, breads, buns, pastries, doughnuts, cookies, ketchup, and ice cream.

Many people unwittingly eat sugar with every meal: breakfast cereals are frosted with sugar, break time is soda or coffee mixed with sugar and a Danish, lunch has its cookies and treats, and dinner could be sweet-and-sour ribs topped off with a sugary dessert. All those sweets can turn your health sour! A U.S. Department of Agriculture study in 2000 revealed that we eat an average of *thirty-two teaspoons* of sugar daily.

Many drink their sugar in the form of Cokes, Pepsis, 7-Ups, and Mountain Dews. Teen boys chug an average of three twelve-ounce cans of soft drinks daily, which contain forty grams of sugar in each drink. Teen girls are just behind at two cans a day,[2] which does not bode well for those with pre-diabetes or undiagnosed diabetes. A Harvard University study demonstrated that drinking more than one sugar-sweetened soft drink a day appears to significantly increase a woman's chances of developing diabetes. The greater risk comes from soda's excess calories and large amount of rapidly absorbable sugars, which send blood glucose levels soaring off the chart.[3]

The Great Physician's Rx for Diabetes calls for eating healthy proteins, healthy fats, and lower amounts of carbohydrates (sugars and starches). The combinations of foods you eat are important as well. I do not recommend that you eat fruit on its own because of its high sugar content; fruit should be consumed with fats and proteins, which will slow down the absorption of sugar.

STARCHY CARBS

Let's turn our attention to the starch side of carbohydrates. When carbohydrates are eaten, the digestive tract breaks down the long chains of starches into single sugars, mainly glucose, which is a source of immediate energy. As mentioned earlier, if these calories are not expended through physical effort, the body converts them to fat, and therein lies a weighty problem. As a culture, we are a little taller but a lot heavier than we were a generation ago; today we weigh twenty-five pounds more than our grandparents or parents did in the 1960s, with the biggest weight gains attached to men forty and older.

A trio of low-carb weight-loss plans—Atkins, South Beach, and Zone—have been flying off the shelf for years, with the *Atkins New Diet Revolution* spending an incredible six years on the *New York Times* bestseller's list. The main premise behind low-carb diets is that reducing the intake of carbohydrates like bread, pasta, and rice reduces insulin levels and causes your body to burn excess body fat for fuel.

My biggest beef with low-carb diets is that most of these health plans advocate a high consumption of meat products that God calls unclean (as I'll explain shortly), allow only limited amounts of nutrient-rich fruits and vegetables, and encourage the consumption of artificial sweeteners and preservatives.

Those with diabetes lean heavily on artificial sweeteners like aspartame-based NutraSweet or Equal, saccharin-based Sweet 'N Low, and chlorinated sucrose-based Splenda. Regarding Splenda, the chemical process to turn sugar into sucralose alters the chemical composition of sugar so much that it is converted into a fructo-galactose molecule. This type of sugar does not occur in nature, which means your body does not possess the ability to properly metabolize it.[4] It's my view that any artificial sweeteners should be treated as toxic substances to the body; they are not the answer for diabetics looking to sweeten their iced tea.

A BETTER ROAD TO HEALTH

I believe in a lower carbohydrate approach to treating diabetes and losing weight. The carbohydrates you want to consume are low glycemic, high nutrient, and low sugar. These would be most high-fiber fruits, especially berries; vegetables; nuts; seeds; and legumes; plus a small amount of whole grain products, which are always better than refined carbohydrates that have been stripped of their vital fiber, vitamin, and mineral components.

Eating unrefined carbohydrate foods, on the other hand, introduces fiber-rich foods into your body. Fiber is the indigestible remnant of plant cells found in vegetables, fruits, whole grains, nuts, seeds, and beans. Fiber-rich foods take longer to break down and are partially indigestible, which means that as these foods work their way through the digestive tract, they absorb water and increase the elimination of waste matter from the large intestine.

Good sources of fiber are berries, fruits with edible skins (apples, pears, and grapes), citrus fruits, whole grains (quinoa, millet, amaranth, buckwheat, and brown rice), green peas, carrots, cucumbers, zucchini, tomatoes, and baked or boiled unpeeled potatoes. Green leafy vegetables such as spinach are also fiber rich. Eating foods high in fiber will immediately improve your blood sugar levels by slowing the absorption of sugars into your bloodstream.

Chewing your food well will also slow the absorption of sugars into your bloodstream. If people tease you about "inhaling" your food, then you're eating too fast. I recommend chewing each mouthful of food twenty-five to seventy-five times before swallowing. This advice may sound ridiculous, but I know that a conscious effort to chew food slowly ensures that plenty of digestive juices are added to the food as it begins to wind through the digestive tract, and that's important for diabetics.

THE IMPORTANCE OF HYDRATION

While you're taking your time to chew your food, be sure to drink plenty of water during *and* in between your meals. Water performs many vital tasks for the body: regulating the body temperature, carrying nutrients and oxygen to the cells, cushioning joints, protecting organs and tissue, and removing toxins. Water happens to be the perfect fluid replacement; only God could come up with a calorie-free and sugar-free substance that makes up 92 percent of your blood plasma and 50 percent of everything else in the body.

F. Batmanghelidj, M.D. and author of *You're Not Sick, You're Thirsty!*, contends that diabetes "seems to be the end result of water deficiency to the brain" because the brain depends on glucose— blood sugar—as a source of energy. If you don't drink enough water, the kidneys can't function properly either. When the body is properly hydrated, however, the kidneys function normally, and the liver converts stored fat into usable energy. In other words, the liver—acting like a traffic cop—will direct the body to tap into its fat reserves when you're eating leaner foods, consuming less calories, and exercising regularly. You can greatly accelerate the liver's ability to convert stored fat into usable energy by consuming an abundance of clean, healthy water.

The importance of staying well hydrated cannot be emphasized enough. Dr. Batmanghelidj believes that many diabetics confuse hunger and thirst, thinking they're hungry when actually they're dehydrated. You should be drinking, at a minimum, at least eight glasses of water each day, which will give the body's vital organs the fluids they need as well as put a damper on the hunger pangs coming from the pit of your stomach.

If you're overweight, downing a glass of water a half hour before lunch or dinner will act like a governor on an engine, taking the edge off your hunger pangs and preventing you from raiding the fridge or pillaging the pantry. "You will feel full and will eat only when food is needed," Dr. Batmanghelidj says. "The volume of food intake will decrease drastically. The type of cravings for food will also change. With sufficient water intake, we tend to crave proteins more than carbohydrates. If you think you are different and your body does not need eight to ten glasses of water each day, you are making a major mistake," he said.[5]

Sure, you'll go to the bathroom more often, but is that so bad? Drinking plenty of water is not only healthy for the body, but it's a key part of the Great Physician's Rx for Diabetes Battle

Plan (see page 73), so keep a water bottle close by and drink water before and during meals.

Coffee Break

Speaking of something to drink, is this country's obsession with Starbucks coffee healthy? Many health experts disagree about whether consuming caffeinated beverages such as coffee or tea is a good idea, but I must point out that coffee and tea have been consumed for thousands of years by some of the world's healthiest people. Although I'm not a huge fan of coffee or a coffee drinker myself, I will say that fresh ground organic coffee flavored with organic cream and honey is fine when consumed in moderation, meaning one cup per day. Teas and herbal infusions (the latter beverage is made from herbs and spices, rather than the actual tea plant) are another story all together.

Infusions of herbs and spices such as teas have been a part of nearly every culture throughout history. In fact, consuming organic teas and herbal infusions several times per day can be one of the best things you can do for your health. Green and white teas, for example, provide the body with antioxidants such as polyphenols, which help reduce cellular damage and oxidative stress. Studies have identified the anticancer compounds in tea as well as compounds that help increase metabolism. Teas and herbal infusions can provide energy, enhance the immune system, improve the digestion, and even help you wind down after a long day.

As far as caffeine is concerned, I believe that teas' benefits are better delivered in teas containing caffeine. Since tea leaves naturally contain caffeine, the Creator obviously intended for us to consume tea in its most natural form. Obviously, if caffeine tends to keep you up at night, you should avoid consuming caffeinated teas in the late afternoon or in the evening. For an after-dinner treat, try consuming a caffeine-free herbal infusion containing relaxing herbs and spices to help you wind down and decompress.

My favorite tea blends contain combinations of tea (green, black, or white) with biblical herbs and spices such as grape, pomegranate, hyssop, olive, and fig leaves. Even though I've never thought of myself as a tea-drinking type, my wife, Nicki, and I enjoy these biblical tea blends with dinner.

You'll find in my Great Physician's Rx for Diabetes Battle Plan (see page 73) that I recommend a cup of hot tea and honey with breakfast, dinner, and snacks. I also advise consuming freshly made iced tea, as tea can be consumed hot or steeped and iced. Please note that while herbal tea provides many great health benefits, nothing can replace pure water for hydration. Although you can safely and healthfully consume two to four cups per day of tea and herbal infusions, you still need to drink at least six cups of pure water for all the good reasons I've described in this chapter.

IF YOU GET THE URGE TO CHEAT

Let's say you're invited to a Super Bowl party. Tables are piled high with tantalizing hors d'oeuvres, crispy finger foods, and tempting sweets. You indulge. You graze. You keep on eating.

You're cheating. Your blood sugar levels are spinning like a slot machine.

How can you minimize the damage? According to Richard and Rachael Heller, authors of *The Carbohydrate Addict's Diet* (Signet, 1993), if you're going to cheat, then get it over with in a one-hour time frame. The Hellers say that when the body has been deprived of insulin-releasing foods high in carbohydrates, the body makes an adjustment. In other words, when you eat during one sixty-minute time frame, the body can be triggered to produce only so much insulin. Continue to snack longer—like right into the second half of the big game—and the body releases a second phase of insulin. That's not good when you have diabetes.

The Hellers advise that when you know you will be put in a situation that may sabotage your desire to eat well and control your diabetes, you should make sure that you eat a healthy, low-carb breakfast and lunch loaded with healthy protein, fat, fruits, and vegetables. When you're at the event, set your clock for one hour, and eat to your heart's content. During that hour, I would strongly recommend that you avoid consuming the worst of the "Dirty Dozen" (see page 22); other than that, you can "release the hounds," but only for that one-hour period.

In addition to the urge to cheat, diabetics often have to deal with food cravings. An efficient way to dampen cravings is to eat foods that aid the body's production of serotonin, a neurotransmitter that gives you a feeling of well-being. Foods known to help the body produce serotonin are cottage cheese, milk, cheese, chicken, turkey, duck, and sesame seeds.

NUTRITION IN A BAR

In an effort to eat healthy and lose weight, many Americans have turned to consuming energy bars as a convenient meal replacement or an in-between snack. Doing this may sound like a good idea, but in reality, many energy bars are no healthier than a handful of Tootsie Rolls. In fact many energy bars contain harmful ingredients such as artificial sweeteners, chemicals, preservatives, and synthetic nutrients.

If you find it difficult to sit down to a home-cooked healthy breakfast every morning, or if you find yourself frequenting the vending machines during snack breaks, you can eat a healthy whole food bar as a meal replacement, healthy snack, or afternoon pick-me-up. In my quest for providing others with healthy alternatives, I've developed one of the finest organic whole food bars available today, containing recommended amounts of protein, omega-3 fats, fiber, and probiotics, along with compounds known as beta-glucans from soluble oat fiber. If you find it difficult to stay away from treats in the employee break room, then check out these whole food bars. (For more information, visit www.BiblicalHealthInstitute.com and click on the GPRx Resource Guide.)

THE TOP HEALING FOODS

We've discussed many healthy foods in this chapter so far, but the following foods are musts for your diet. In addition, keep this in mind when you sit down to eat: you should consume the protein, fats, and vegetables first before swallowing any fruit, sweeteners, or high-starch carbohydrates like potatoes, rice, grains, and bread. I know it's hard to resist fresh bread when it's presented in a nice restaurant, but you would be better off having a piece toward the end of your meal.

1. Wild-caught Fish

Fish caught in the wild are a richer source of omega-3 fats, protein, potassium, vitamins, and minerals than farm-raised fish, which are kept in cement ponds and fed a diet of food pellets. You can purchase fresh salmon and other wild-caught fish from your local fish market or health food store. Many other fish are healthy as well, including sardines, herring, mackerel, tuna, snapper, bass, and cod.

2. Cultured Dairy Products from Goats, Cows, and Sheep

Dairy products derived from goat's milk and sheep's milk can be healthier for some individuals than those from cows, although dairy products from organic or grass-fed cows can be excellent as well. Goat's milk is less allergenic because it does not contain the same complex proteins found in cow's milk.

I do not recommend drinking 2 percent or skim milk because removing the fat makes the milk less nutritious and less digestible, and it can cause allergies. Yes, whole milk has more calories, but this is not an area to cut corners. I've seen research suggesting that the mix of nutrients found in milk, such as calcium and protein, may improve the body's ability to burn fat, particularly around the midsection.

3. A Wide Selection of Fruits and Vegetables

Nutritionists have long known that fruits and vegetables are low in calories and high in fiber content. As mentioned earlier, eating plenty of fruits and vegetables—five servings a day are recommended—benefits those wanting to lose weight.

I've described how fruits and vegetables satisfy your hunger with fewer calories. You're going to save hundreds of calories a day by substituting sweets with just-as-sweet in-season fruits. Many fruits and vegetables are high in water, which provides volume in the pit of your stomach, not calories. Since these high-fiber foods take longer to digest, you feel full longer. It's kind of like having gastric bypass surgery without all the nasty side effects.

4. Soaked and Sprouted Seeds and Grains

Like fruits and vegetables, sprouted grains, seeds, nuts, and whole grains are high in fiber. *Whole grain* means the bran and germ are left on the grain during processing. *Soaked grains* retain their plant enzymes when they are not cooked. This process greatly helps digestion.

5. Cultured and Fermented Vegetables

Often greeted with upturned noses at the dinner table, fermented vegetables such as sauerkraut, pickled carrots, beets, or cucumbers are overlooked by those on a diet, even though they are some of the healthiest foods on the planet. Raw cultured or fermented vegetables supply the body with useful organisms known as probiotics, as well as many vitamins, including vitamin C.

If you've never put a fork on any of these foods before, I urge you to sample sauerkraut or pickled beets, which are readily available in health food stores.

6. Healthy Fats

Foods high in healthy fats, including olives, avocados, nuts and seeds and their butters, olive oil, flaxseed oil, coconut oil, and butter produced from healthy animals, can be wonderful allies in your quest for weight loss. Extra virgin coconut oil has been the recipient of some great press the last few years for its ability to help balance the thyroid, aid in metabolism, and assist with energy production. Some experts recommend that people with thyroid and weight troubles should consume as many as two to four tablespoons of coconut oil per day. Make sure to consume healthy fats with every meal to provide satiety and slow the absorption of sugar into the bloodstream, thereby keeping blood sugar and insulin levels at an even keel.

A balanced thyroid plays a vital role in your metabolism. Mary Shomon, author of *The Thyroid Diet* (Collins, 2004), says that certain foods high in tyrosine assist the body in the production of the thyroid hormone T3, which helps you utilize more oxygen and burn more calories. Foods high in tyrosine are cottage cheese, egg whites, safflower seeds, and meats such as turkey, antelope, quail, and buffalo.

7. Herbs and Spices

The use of herbs (rather than rich sauces on meats) and spices (rather than dressings, creams, or oil) is an excellent strategy for weight loss. I'm not talking about dousing your food in table salt, which is high in sodium, but employing strong flavors such as garlic, chili powder, cayenne, curry powder, rosemary, and tarragon to add taste to the foods you eat. A particularly beneficial culinary spice for improving diabetes is cinnamon because of its ability to reestablish insulin sensitivity, which is significantly decreased by diabetes.

A chemical in cinnamon, called methylhydroxy chalcone polymer (MHCP), has been shown to increase glucose metabolism of fat cells twentyfold, according to research findings from the Human Nutrition Research Center, a branch of the U.S. Department of Agriculture. Researchers at the Beltsville Human Nutrition Research Center in Maryland gave sixty people with type 2 diabetes various amounts of cinnamon every day for forty days, while those in a control group were handed placebos. People receiving half a teaspoon of cinnamon daily experienced a drop in blood sugar, fat, and cholesterol levels by as much as 30 percent.[6] Researchers believe that cinnamon may delay the onset of type 2 diabetes for those at risk.

Since cinnamon is proving to be a wonderful spice for blood sugar levels, I recommend that you sprinkle cinnamon on a piece of toast or in a smoothie or even mixed with cottage cheese, honey, and raisins every day. If you're diabetic, you should incorporate between a quarter teaspoon and one teaspoon into your daily diet.

THE DIRTY DOZEN

Whether you're diagnosed with diabetes or not, there are certain foods that should never find a way onto your plate or into your hands. Here are what I call the Dirty Dozen:

1. *Pork products.* In all of my books, I've consistently pointed out that pork—America's "other white meat"—should be avoided because pigs were called "unclean" in Leviticus and Exodus. God labeled certain animals, birds, and fish "unclean" because they are scavengers who feed off trash—or worse.

2. *Shellfish and fish without fins and scales, such as catfish, shark, and eel.* In the Old Testament, God called hard-shelled crustaceans such as lobsters, crabs, and clams unclean as well. Their flesh harbors known toxins that can contribute to poor health.

3. *Hydrogenated oils.* Margarine and shortening are taboo.

4. *Artificial sweeteners.* Diabetics who can't drink Pepsi or Coke straight up often turn to diet versions sweetened with aspartame, saccharin, and sucralose, to name a few. Yet these artificial sweeteners are made from chemicals, and their safety has sparked debate for decades.

5. *White flour.* One thing we've learned over the years: enriched white flour is not a diabetic's best friend.

6. *White sugar.* If you're looking for a culprit to blame for the diabetes epidemic, then look no further.

7. *Soft drinks.* Run, don't hide, from this liquefied sugar. A twelve-ounce Coke or Pepsi is the equivalent of eating nearly nine teaspoons of sugar.

8. *Pasteurized homogenized skim milk.* Like I said, whole organic milk is better, and goat's milk is best.

9. *Corn syrup.* This is another version of sugar and even more fattening.

10. *Hydrolyzed soy protein.* If you're wondering what in the world this is, hydrolyzed soy protein is found in imitation meat products. Stick to the real stuff.

11. *Artificial flavors and colors.* These are never good for you under the best of circumstances, and certainly not when you're trying to lose weight.

12. *Excessive alcohol.* Although studies point out the benefits of drinking small amounts of red wine for the heart (part of the "French paradox"), the fact remains that alcohol contains lots of calories. Overconsumption of alcohol has wrecked millions of families over the years.

EAT: WHAT FOODS ARE EXTRAORDINARY, AVERAGE, OR TROUBLE?

I've prepared a comprehensive list of foods that are ranked in descending order based on their health-giving qualities. Foods at the top of the list are healthier than those at the bottom. When eating, practice portion control. Put less food on your plate than you usually do and see what happens. A Pennsylvania State University study found that reducing serving size by 25 percent can help you consume up to 800 fewer calories per day without reducing satisfaction.[7]

The best foods to serve and eat are what I call extraordinary, which God created for us to eat and are in a form healthy for the body. If you are struggling with your blood sugar and weight, it is best to consume foods from the Extraordinary category more than 75 percent of the time.

Foods in the Average category should make up less then 50 percent of your daily diet. If you are struggling with your weight, it's best to limit consumption of average foods to less than 25 percent of your daily diet.

Foods in the Trouble category do not promote weight loss and should be consumed with extreme caution. If you are trying to lose weight, you should avoid these foods completely.

For a complete listing of Extraordinary, Average, and Trouble Foods, visit www.BiblicalHealthInstitute.com/EAT.

Foods in the Trouble category do not promote weight loss and should be consumed with extreme caution. If you are trying to lose weight, you should avoid these foods completely.

For a listing of Extraordinary, Average, and Trouble Foods, visit www.BiblicalHealthInstitute.com/EAT.

℞ THE GREAT PHYSICIAN'S Rx FOR DIABETES: EAT TO LIVE

- *Eat only foods God created.*

- *Eat foods in a form that is healthy for the body.*

- *At mealtime, consume protein, fat, and veggies before sweets or starchy carbohydrates.*

- *Practice portion control by putting 20 percent less on your plate.*

- *Drink six to eight or more glasses of pure water per day, and drink eight ounces of water whenever you feel hungry.*

- *When the food on your plate is half-eaten, take a deep breath and ask yourself if you're still hungry.*

- *Eat foods like whole oatmeal or whole food nutrition bars, which contain beta-glucans.*

- *Sprinkle between a quarter teaspoon and a teaspoon of cinnamon daily into your foods.*

Take Action

To learn how to incorporate the principles of eating to live into your daily regimen, please turn to page 73 for the Great Physician's Rx for Diabetes Battle Plan.

KEY #2

Supplement Your Diet with Whole Food Nutritionals, Living Nutrients, and Superfoods

I don't see how people with type 2 diabetes can optimize their health without using nutritional supplements. My reasoning goes like this: because the body breaks down food to gain energy and nutrients, most of those with type 2 diabetes have gunked up the works through poor diet, lack of exercise, and consumption of too many foods with sugar. While my first key, "Eat to live," is a solid punch against diabetes, supplementing your diet with whole food nutritionals, living nutrients, and superfoods can knock this disease out of the ring.

I speak from experience because I began taking whole food supplements, along with probiotics and enzymes, when I was at my sickest. Once I ingested the right supplements (I had previously taken hundreds of the wrong ones), I noticed an immediate improvement in my health problems, including the color of my legs, which were purple from the lack of blood circulation and nutrients in my blood. Since then, I have a Cal Ripken streak going: I've taken nutritional supplements *every day* for more than a decade. That's at least 3,650 consecutive days for those of you keeping score at home.

Let me tell you about an average day for me. Whenever I sit down for a meal, I discreetly reach for a silver case and pop it open. I pick out a few whole food living multivitamins and a couple of "live" probiotic and enzyme capsules, and I wash them down with a glass of water. Later on during the day, I ingest a green food/fiber blend supplement. My "chaser" is a heaping spoonful of one of my absolute favorite supplements—omega-3 cod-liver oil.

Some of you may be suppressing a gag reflex, but my reason for taking this wide array of nutritional supplements is not because I fail to eat healthy. My wife, Nicki, is a wonderful cook armed with dozens of fantastic recipes built around free-range or wild meats, organic vegetables, healthy oils, and fresh fruits.

Because I travel a great deal, there are times when I find myself in settings where I'm served meals that aren't the highest quality. I think it's a fair statement to say that the typical American diet strays from God's design with its glamorous array of mass-produced foods replete with empty calories, refined carbohydrates, and woefully inadequate nutrition. Taking whole food nutritional supplements covers my bases and offers a concentrated source of nutrients that plant foods don't always provide, mainly because of depletions in nutrient-barren soils.

Back in biblical times, foods coming from the fields contained many more vitamins, minerals, enzymes, and beneficial microorganisms than what's sold in supermarkets today. For the past half century or so, we've been sterilizing our soil with pesticides and herbicides, using synthetic fertilizers, and not letting our fields lay fallow every seven years as God commanded, which means our food—even what is organically grown—doesn't pack the same nutritional punch as it did for our forefathers.

From the outset, though, please know that I'm not one who believes type 2 diabetes can be turned around with a bottle of pills. After years of study in naturopathic medicine and nutrition, I understand better than most that dietary supplements are just what they say they are—supplements, not substitutes for an inadequate diet and unhealthy lifestyle.

STARTING YOUR DAY OFF RIGHT

When I talk to diabetics about supplementing their diets, I begin with multivitamins, and I have good news to report about them. In a double-blind study, middle-aged and elderly diabetics who took a multiple vitamin and mineral preparation for one year avoided respiratory and gastrointestinal infections by more than 80 percent, as compared to those diabetics given a placebo.[1] Dr. Thomas Barringer, director of research at Carolinas Medical Center in Charlotte, North Carolina, said that diabetes can leave people prone to infections because out-of-control blood sugar compromises the immune system and leads to minor deficiencies of certain minerals that are lost in excessive urination.

Multivitamins play a role in preventing diabetes because certain ingredients—chromium, vanadium, and magnesium—promote healthier blood sugar levels. Chromium and vanadium mimic insulin and help the body produce more of the hormone. As for magnesium, scientists believe that the mineral gives the pancreas the nutrients it needs to produce insulin. The study of chromium, vanadium, and magnesium and their relationship to diabetes is not fully understood, but scientists are confident that this trio of nutrients can improve diabetes control.

While researchers continue their work, I'm confident that those with diabetes will greatly benefit from taking a quality whole food multivitamin that supplies highly bioavailable nutrients in proper balance. Multivitamin supplements are especially important to overweight diabetics because many obese individuals are nutritionally deficient, and the stress from dealing with diabetes day in and day out can deplete the body of certain nutrients.

The American Diabetes Association, on its Web site, referred to a study performed at Shaheed Beheshti University of Medical Sciences in Tehran, Iran, of all places. The researchers divided the type 2 diabetes study members into four groups:

1. One group was given zinc sulfate and magnesium oxide.
2. One group received vitamin C and vitamin E.
3. One group received all four vitamins and minerals: zinc sulfate, magnesium oxide, vitamin C, and vitamin E.
4. One group received a placebo each day.

After three months it turned out that the group taking all *four* vitamins and minerals (zinc sulfate, magnesium oxide, vitamin C, and vitamin E) experienced the greatest reduction in blood pressure, which eased some of their symptoms for diabetes.

A good whole food multivitamin contains many more ingredients than zinc, magnesium, vitamin C, and vitamin E. These types of vitamins contain different compounds such as organic acids, antioxidants, and key nutrients, which are all essential to good health. They are more costly to produce since the ingredients— fruits, vegetables, sea vegetables, seeds, spices, vitamins and minerals, and so on—are put through a fermentation process similar to the digestive process of the body, but they are well worth the extra money.

The *best* multivitamins are produced from raw materials by adding vitamins and minerals to a living probiotic culture. If you're scratching your head and saying, "Huh?" let me explain. Multivitamins are produced several different ways. Some are derived from vegetable, mineral, or animal sources such as cod-liver oil, wheat germ oil, or yeast. Other multivitamins are derived from processing that extracts vitamins from fish liver oil, soybeans, and other natural sources.

The most common form of multivitamins, however, is synthetically produced in a chemist's lab and is also the cheapest to produce. If you see ingredients such as sucrose, cornstarch, thiamine mononitrate, pyridoxine hydrochloride, ascorbic acid, or sodium metasilicate listed, your multivitamin is produced from synthetic materials. Synthetic multivitamins are never going to be as good or potent as ones produced from natural sources; studies show that synthetically made vitamins are 50 to 70 percent less biologically active than vitamins created from natural sources. Another giveaway is seeing the letters *dl* in front of the name of an ingredient. An ingredient named dl-alpha tocopheryl, for example, informs you that you're taking a synthetic version of vitamin E.

If you're currently on medication for diabetes, research suggests that you may be deficient in folic acid and vitamin B_{12}, which should be contained in your whole food nutritional supplements. Besides giving you nutrients in good balance, a quality whole food multivitamin contains certain minerals—chromium, magnesium, and vanadium—that help to balance blood sugar levels, which improves metabolism.

Whole food multivitamins also cover your bases because our food isn't as nutritious as it used to be because of soil depletion. These multivitamins come packaged in different varieties: tablets and capsules are the most common; powders and liquids are less widespread. I prefer caplets as a good delivery system to ensure the nutrients get where they need to go.

OPEN UP TO COD-LIVER OIL

Those with type 2 diabetes not only have high levels of fat in their blood, but they also travel through life with low levels of HDL, the "good" cholesterol. Doctors in Denmark discovered that sipping spoonfuls of fish liver oil daily helps those with type 2 diabetes slash the high levels of fat—known as triglycerides—in their blood cells. I must point out, however, that results of eighteen trials over a ten-year period show that while fish oil lowers triglycerides, the supplement appears to have no statistically significant effect on glycemic (blood sugar) control.[2]

The best type of fish oil to add to your daily nutritional regime is omega-3 cod liver oil extracted from cod taken from the freezing waters of the North Atlantic. Cod-liver oil is one of the best sources for omega-3 fatty acids known to man—an extraordinary nutritional resource that has been acknowledged to play a leading role in the development of the brain, the rods and cones of the retina of the eye, the lubrication of the joints, and the body's inflammatory response. Omega-3 fatty acids are beneficial to those suffering from diabetes and obesity. Besides decreasing cholesterol and triglyceride levels, omega-3 fatty acids lower blood pressure and appear to have antidepressant and mood-stabilizing effects.

The golden oils extracted from the filleted livers of Icelandic cod may be an acquired taste, but after a decade of sipping spoonfuls of cod-liver oil, I'm at the point where I can drink the stuff right out of the bottle. If you can't "stomach" the thought of sipping omega-3 cod-liver oil, you can now take this important nutrient in easy-to-swallow liquid capsules. (For recommended products, visit www.BiblicalHealthInstitute.com and click on the GPRx Resource Guide.)

GREEN FOODS

I would hazard a guess that if you have diabetes, then you're not a big vegetable eater—especially the green leafy kind. If you're having trouble motivating yourself to eat your veggies, I know a way your body can receive more green foods, which contain nutrients not found in the typical low-carbohydrate diet. I recommend the consumption of green superfood powders and caplets. All you do is mix the powder in water or your favorite juice, or swallow a handful of caplets.

A good green food supplement is a certified organic blend of dried green vegetables, fermented vegetables, sea vegetables, microalgaes such as spirulina and chlorella, and sprouted grains and seeds. When you drink or swallow green foods, your body is taking in one of the most nutrient-dense foods on this green earth—but containing less than one-twentieth the calories of a Big Mac value meal.

This is what I call a real two-fer: not only is a green food supplement high in nutrients and low in calories, but it gives you the dietary benefits of whole food living nutrients, including improving digestion and elimination.

WHOLE FOOD FIBER BLEND

As mentioned in Key #1, fiber can be a diabetic's best friend. Consuming adequate fiber will ensure a feeling of satiety since fiber delays the absorption of sugars in the body and provides a sense of fullness. An additional benefit is that fiber improves regularity, which helps to efficiently eliminate toxins from the body. Since most of us get about one-fifth of the optimal amount of fiber in our daily diet, I recommend taking a whole food fiber supplement. Look for one that supplies your body with a highly usable, vegetarian source of dietary fiber.

When searching for a fiber product that's right for you, choose a brand made from organic seeds, grains, and legumes that are fermented or sprouted for ease of digestion. One of the preferred ways to consume whole food fiber is to take a combination green superfood/fiber blend first thing in the morning and just before bed—mix it with your favorite juice or water. When you do, you're giving your body more nutrition than most people get in a week while promoting maintenance of healthy blood sugar levels. (For a list of recommended whole food fiber products, visit www.BiblicalHealthInstitute.com and click on the GPRx Resource Guide.)

PROBIOTICS

By definition, probiotics are living, direct-fed microbials, or DFMs, which promote the growth of beneficial or "friendly" bacteria in the intestinal tract. Many diabetic people have digestive problems because they put around-the-clock pressure on the gut to digest everything coming its way, or they eat the *wrong* foods, such as unclean meats drizzled with rich sauces, processed snack foods, or icky-sweet desserts.

When I was attending Florida State University, I was sicker than a Georgia bulldog for a host of intestinal ailments, including the runs. After I introduced whole food probiotics into my system, my health improved immensely. What happens is that the probiotics crowd out disease-causing bacteria, viruses, and yeasts. If you're experiencing constant intestinal pain, then supplement your diet with probiotics. The most effective probiotics contain soil-based organisms (SBOs), multiple strains of lactobacillus and bifidobacteria, and the friendly yeast saccharomyces boulardii. (For recommended brands, visit www.BiblicalHealthInstitute.com and click on the GPRx Resource Guide.)

ENZYMES

When you eat raw foods such as salad and fruits, you consume the enzymes they contain. When you eat cooked or processed meals, such as those from a restaurant kitchen, however, the body's pancreas must produce the enzymes necessary to digest them. The constant demand for enzymes strains the pancreas, which must kick in more enzymes to keep up with the demand. Without the proper levels of enzymes from foods—either raw or fermented—or from supplements, you are susceptible to excessive gas and bloating, diarrhea, constipation, heartburn, and low energy. Do these symptoms sound familiar?

Digestive enzymes are complex proteins involved in the digestive process. They are the body's day laborers, the ones responsible for synthesizing, delivering, and eliminating the unbelievable number of ingredients and chemicals that your body uses during your waking hours. When your body produces enzymes, their job is to stimulate chemical changes in the foods passing through the gut. The pancreas, which takes a lead role in producing digestive enzymes for the body, has to keep up by producing pancreatic enzymes. Those with pancreatic problems such as cystic fibrosis usually require some form of digestive enzyme, but junk food diets, fast chewing, and eating on the run contribute to the body's inability to produce adequate enzyme production and the subsequent malabsorption of food. These problems get worse as we age, not better.

If you're seeking to minimize the consumption of high-enzyme foods such as bananas, avocados, seeds, and grapes—

which are high in sugars as well—then take plant-based digestive enzymes to ease the digestion of food. (You can find recommended brands by visiting www.BiblicalHealthInstitute.com and clicking on the GPRx Resource Guide.)

PROTEIN POWDER

Maintaining adequate protein levels is important for blood sugar control, which is why some diabetics drink protein powder shakes during the day. Careful, though: protein powders sold in warehouse clubs, drugstores, supermarkets, and even natural food stores are usually derived from soy, milk, or whey protein. These protein powders are highly processed and derived from cows injected with hormones and fed antibiotic grain. If you can decipher the ingredient list, you'll detect artificial sweeteners, flavorings, and additives. You have several healthier options: using a whey protein from grass-fed, free-range cows, a fermented soy protein, or a protein powder made from goat's milk.

FINAL THOUGHT

There is no doubt in my mind that the right amount of high-quality whole food nutritional supplements will make a big difference in your diabetes. However, keep in mind that the term *supplement* means "in addition to," so I want to encourage you to base your health plan on eating healthy, organic food and using supplements such as whole food multivitamins, omega-3 cod-liver oil, green superfoods, whole food fiber, enzymes, probiotics, and high-quality protein powders to aid in your quest for a long and healthy life.

℞ THE GREAT PHYSICIAN'S RX FOR DIABETES: SUPPLEMENT YOUR DIET

- *Take a whole food living multivitamin with each meal.*

- *Consume one to three teaspoons or three to nine capsules of omega-3 cod-liver oil per day.*

- *Take a whole food fiber/green food blend with beta-glucans from soluble oat fiber twice per day (morning and evening).*

- *Take an antioxidant/energy product with B vitamins, folic acid, and chromium with each meal.*

- *If you want improved digestion, take enzymes and probiotics.*

- *To ensure optimal protein intake, incorporate an easily digestible protein powder into your daily diet.*

Take Action

To learn how to incorporate the principles of supplementing your diet with whole food nutritionals, living
nutrients, and superfoods into your daily regimen,
please turn to page 73 for the Great Physician's Rx for
Diabetes Battle Plan.

KEY #3

Practice Advanced Hygiene

All patients with diabetes must have a higher standard of hygiene if they are to control repeated infections and other immune system problems," wrote Kenneth Seaton, Ph.D., a pioneer in advanced hygiene and immune system regulation. Dr. Seaton, the author of *Life, Health, and Longevity* (Scientific Hygiene, 1994), believes improved hygiene—along with nutrition and exercise—are the principal ingredients for turning around the health of those with type 2 diabetes. Taking preventive measures against infections, especially during periods of high blood sugar, is very important.

I became aware of Dr. Seaton and his groundbreaking work when I was recuperating from my own serious health challenges. Dr. Seaton had discovered that ear, nose, and throat problems, which represent 80 percent of visits to doctors' offices, could be linked to how we touch our noses, eyes, mouths, and skin with dirty fingernails throughout the day. When we touch ourselves with our hands, we inoculate ourselves with germs that can enter the body through the mouth, a nasal passageway, or the corner of the eyes.

Dr. Seaton is an Australian microbiologist who lives with his family in the United States. He coined the phrase, "Germs don't fly; they hitchhike," after his studies powerfully demonstrated that germs were more likely to be spread by hand-to-hand contact as opposed to airborne exposure. If you want to remain in good health, keep the areas underneath the fingernails, around the membranes of the eyes, and in the front part of the nasal passageway as clean as possible. This information is particularly relevant to those with diabetes because your immune system may have been severely affected by the disease.

Those with diabetes may not be aware that the disease also weakens the mouth's germ-fighting abilities. High blood sugar levels worsen gum disease, and gum disease makes diabetes harder to control. Gum disease is estimated to happen three times more frequently in diabetic patients who have elevated blood sugar levels than those without diabetes.[1] The following are warning signs to look for:

- red, swollen, or tender gums, especially after brushing or flossing your teeth
- gums that have pulled away from the teeth, exposing part of the tooth's root
- oozing pus when you press on the gums (although it would seem hard not to notice this)
- loose teeth moving away from each other

Oral infections are another manifestation of diabetes. When clusters of germs cause problems in one area of your mouth, you should seek medical and dental attention.

But you can take steps to avoid reaching that point by practicing advanced hygiene.

A PRIMER ON GERMS

How do you get germs on your hands? By shaking hands with others or touching things they touched: handrails, doorknobs, shopping carts, paper money, coins, and food. Whenever you read about a breakout of E. coli infections, you can bet your last dollar that it can be traced to a restaurant where workers and cooks who were tossing salads and handling food didn't wash their hands after using the bathroom.

I know this stuff isn't pleasant dinnertime conversation, but hygiene is part of the Great Physician's prescription for health and wellness, which is why I've been following an advanced hygiene protocol for more than a decade with startling results in my life: no lingering head colds, no nagging sinus infections, and no acute respiratory illnesses to speak of for many years.

Here's what I do: each morning and evening, I dip both hands into a tub of semisoft soap and dig my fingernails into the cream. Then I work the special cream soap around the tips of my fingers, cuticles, and fingernails for fifteen to thirty seconds. When I'm finished, I lather my hands for fifteen seconds before rinsing them under running water. After my hands are clean, I take another dab of semisoft soap and wash my face.

My second step involves a procedure that I call a facial dip. I fill my washbasin or a clean, large bowl with warm but not hot water. When enough water is in the basin, I add one or two table-spoons of regular table salt and two eyedroppers of a mineral-based facial solution into the cloudy water. I mix everything with my hands, and then I bend over and dip my face into the cleansing matter, opening my eyes several times to allow the membranes to be cleaned. After coming up for air, I dunk my head a second time and blow bubbles through my nose. "Sink snorkeling," I call it.

My final two steps of advanced hygiene involve applying very diluted drops of hydrogen peroxide and minerals into my ears for thirty to sixty seconds to cleanse the ear canals, and brushing my teeth with an essential oil-based tooth solution to cleanse my mouth of unhealthy germs.

Following this advanced hygiene protocol involves discipline; you have to remind yourself to do it until it becomes an ingrained habit. I find it easier to follow these steps in the morning and before bed. Since starting my hygiene regimen, I just don't feel clean without it. And the best part is, it takes less than three minutes from start to finish.

I urge you to incorporate advanced hygiene into your life, paying special attention to washing your hands periodically, especially after you've been in public situations and shaken the hands of a few friends. I don't want to drive up anyone's paranoia meter, but sometimes our biggest exposure to germs all week happens after church, when we're shaking hands with old friends and new acquaintances in the foyer. All the while, we're exchanging a garden variety of bacteria, allergens, environmental toxins, and viruses from one part of the body to another. So wash those hands well—and often.

Rx THE GREAT PHYSICIAN'S Rx FOR DIABETES: PRACTICE ADVANCED HYGIENE

- *Wash your hands regularly, paying special attention to removing germs from underneath your fingernails.*

- *Cleanse your nasal passageways and the mucous membranes of the eyes daily by performing a facial dip.*

- *Cleanse the ear canals at least twice per week.*

- *Use an essential oil–based tooth solution daily to remove germs from the mouth and improve the health of the gums.*

Take Action

To learn how to incorporate the principles of practicing advanced hygiene into your daily regimen, please turn to page 73 for the Great Physician's Rx for Diabetes Battle Plan.

KEY #4

Condition Your Body with Exercise and Body Therapies

Ron Cook, a correctional officer who supervised seventy-five deputies at Sedgwick County Jail in Wichita, Kansas, liked to start the day by visiting Squeaky's Doughnuts next door to the county lockup.

I know there's a joke somewhere about a cop and a doughnut shop, but that was Ron's daily routine. He was partial to the buttermilk doughnuts with a sugar glaze, and he enjoyed eating two of them with his sugared coffee. Ron arrived at 5:30 every morning, giving him a chance to hang out with other sheriff's deputies before the start of their shift at 6:00 a.m.

Fifty years old now, Ron was recently forced into retirement because of his diabetic condition. Years of poor diet, lack of sleep, and no exercise had taken its toll on him and his personal life: he's been married four times. So when Ron heard me speak at Central Christian Church in Wichita, he was ready to make major lifestyle changes, including getting enough rest and starting an exercise program.

Getting enough sleep was always difficult for Ron, who carried the stress of running a correctional facility with 1,400 prisoners on his broad shoulders. Most nights, Ron didn't get more than five or six hours of shut-eye, leaving him feeling unrefreshed when the alarm clock jangled him awake at 4:45 a.m.

Ron was among the one hundred million Americans who get

45

up each morning without enough proper rest. The root causes of our national sleep debt are overcrowded schedules, the desire to accomplish one more thing before retiring, and too much stimulation from watching TV. This is a shame because those who sleep less than five hours are 2.5 times more likely to have diabetes, according to a study performed at Boston University.[1] Dr. Daniel Gottlieb, the study's coauthor, said researchers adjusted the statistics to remove any influence of gender, age, race, or body type. According to the study, a lack of rest impairs the body's ability to process glucose, a cause of diabetes. For type 2 diabetics struggling to lose weight, not enough sleep boosts the appetite, especially for high-calorie, high-carbohydrate foods.

Sleep is a major regulator of leptin, a hormone that tells the brain that it doesn't need more food, and ghrelin, a different hormone that triggers hunger. When test subjects slept only four hours nightly, leptin levels decreased by 18 percent, and ghrelin levels increased 28 percent.[2] Translation: they had the munchies for a midnight snack.

Dr. Gottlieb said his study bolstered the common recommendation for sleeping seven or eight hours a night, which I would amend to something closer to eight hours than to seven hours. Eight hours is the number to shoot for because when people can control the amount of time they sleep, such as in a sleep laboratory, they naturally sleep eight hours in a twenty-four-hour period.

Like millions of Americans, my wife, Nicki, and I wish we could catch eight wonderful, blissful hours of sleep, but as parents of an energetic toddler, we've gotten used to getting up in the middle of the night to tend to him. If Joshua is cooperative, we get our eight hours, although as Nicki would remind me, I'm speaking for myself since moms often sleep with one eye open and the other closed.

What I've found most beneficial is following the advice of my friend and colleague Dr. Joseph Mercola of Mercola.com, who told me that one hour of sleep *before* midnight is equal to four hours of sleep *after* midnight. I know Dr. Joe is right because when I go to bed really late, say around 2:00 a.m., I don't feel well in the morning—or the next day. But when I go to bed before midnight, I wake up refreshed and ready to hit the day.

There's More Than Just Sleep

Sleep is just one of a half-dozen body therapies that you should incorporate into your lifestyle. A close cousin to sleep is rest, which also seems to be in short supply these days. We don't get enough rest because of our "shop until you drop" culture that's available 24/7. In the last decade, neighborhood supermarkets have begun to stay open all night long, as have chain pharmacy stores. When the latest Harry Potter books go on sale, bookstores stay open in the middle of the night so they can officially begin selling them at midnight. And shopping online is perfect for someone trying to squeeze in one more purchase that day.

Busy weekends exacerbate the problem. Malls and other shopping emporiums vie for shoppers' dollars with alluring sales, and many families run themselves ragged driving their kids to all the soccer, T-ball, and lacrosse games. Woe to the parents with children good enough to play on travel teams.

Families need a time of rest by taking a break from the rat race on Saturday or Sunday. God created the earth and the heavens in six days and rested on the seventh, giving us an example and a reminder that we need to take a break from our labors. Just as triathletes and other high-performance athletes are careful to give their bodies one day off a week, we should be as well. Otherwise, we're prime candidates for burnout.

GIVE ME TWENTY OR DROP

A body therapy that is just as important to diabetes is exercise. Many who have diabetes are overweight and often obese, and exercise may be as foreign as a Roberto Benigni film. Exercise doeth a body good, whether you're an overweight diabetic or not.

You cannot afford *not* to exercise, and if that means scheduling an appointment with a trainer at a gym, then do so. Trying to control your blood sugar or lose weight without exercising would be like trying to ace a final exam without studying. While it can be done, ninety-nine times out of a hundred you can't lose weight—or at least sustain any weight loss—without stoking the body's furnace to burn up reserves of fat.

Exercise is also key to managing diabetes and blood glucose levels. When you huff and puff, the body demands extra energy (in the form of glucose) for the muscles, which lowers blood glucose levels. Moderate exercise prompts the muscles to ask for glucose at nearly twenty times the normal rate. In addition, when you exercise faithfully, you will

- improve your body's use of insulin.
- burn excess body fat, which results in improved insulin sensitivity.
- improve muscle strength and increase bone density.
- lower blood pressure levels and reduce the risk of heart disease.
- lower "bad" LDL cholesterol levels and increase "good" HDL cholesterol levels.

What kind of exercise should you do when you have diabetes? If the last time you darkened a gym was when George Herbert Walker Bush lived in the White House, I know a great way to get back into the exercise game. It's called *functional fitness,* and this form of gentle exercise will get your body burning calories and improve agility. The idea behind functional fitness is to train movements, not muscles, as you build up cardiovascular endurance and the body's core muscles. You do this through performing real-life activities in real-life positions. (Please visit www.GreatPhysiciansRx.com for in-depth instructions of functional fitness exercises.)

Functional fitness uses body weight exercises, but can also employ dumbbells, mini trampolines, and stability balls. It is gaining popularity around the country. Instructors at LA Fitness, Bally Total Fitness, and local YMCAs put you through a series of exercises that mimic everyday life. You're asked to perform squats with feet apart, feet together, and one back with the other forward. You're asked to do reaching lunges, push-ups against a wall, and "supermans" that involve lying on the floor and lifting up your right arm while lifting your left leg into a fully extended position. What you're *not* asked to perform are high-impact exercises like those found in energetic, pulsating aerobics classes.

A functional fitness program provides an entry-level approach to exercise, increases strength in the daily tasks of life, and when done twice a day for five to fifteen minutes at a time, burns calories so that you can lose unwanted weight.

One surefire way to improve your health is to start walking, which is an excellent form of exercise for those battling diabetes. Walking is a low-impact but surprisingly effective exercise that places a gentle strain on the heart muscle as you work up to better fitness.

Walking around the neighborhood or on a treadmill at a fitness facility can be done when it's most convenient for you. You can walk before work, during your lunch hour, or before dinner. You set the pace; you decide how much to put into this exercise.

If possible, you can kill two birds with one stone by walking in the sunlight. Exposing your face and skin to sunlight is another body therapy I recommend because it gives the body a chance to synthesize vitamin D from the ultraviolet rays of the sun. Getting some sun—whether on a walk or sitting in a chair outside work or in the backyard—has important health ramifications for those with diabetes. The vitamin D in sunlight, when synthesized by the body, augments the production of insulin. When not enough insulin is present in the bloodstream, the body naturally wants to raise insulin levels, and it does that by signaling a hunger for high-carbohydrate foods. Sun exposure will help your metabolism and insulin levels.

I recommend finding at least fifteen minutes of sunlight a day to capture the vitamin D in the rays of the sun. If you're living underneath a gray cloud cover, then take one-to-three teaspoons or three-to-nine capsules of omega-3 cod liver oil daily, which is another important source of vitamin D.

HOT AND COLD IDEAS

In *The Great Physician's Rx for Health and Wellness,* I devoted an entire section to hydrotherapy, aromatherapy, and music therapy. These forms of therapy encourage relaxation, reduce stress, and flush out toxins.

Hydrotherapy comes in the form of baths, showers, washing, and wraps—using hot *and* cold water. For instance, I wake up with a hot shower in the mornings, but then I turn off the hot water and stand under the brisk cold water for about a minute, which totally invigorates me. Cold water stimulates the body and boosts oxygen use in the cells, while hot water dilates blood vessels, which improves blood circulation (important for those with diabetic neuropathy) and transports more oxygen to the brain.

The next time you shower, warm up your body first with hot water. Then slowly turn off the hot water until the cool water becomes cold. Stay under the cold nozzle for at least a minute. You'll feel an increase in energy while improving body awareness.

Hot baths are good for those with diabetes because the hot water on skin expands blood vessels, filling them with blood. Taking a cold or cool shower afterward causes constriction, which improves blood flow. I recommend adding essential oils or herbs to the bath to enhance the therapeutic benefits.

Sitting in a sauna is another form of hydrotherapy. Some with diabetes do not have normal temperature sensation, particularly in their feet, so pay attention. A sauna will not make you lose weight, if that's what you're interested in. Sure, you'll sweat a lot, but any weight loss is likely to be a form of water loss from perspiration. You'll gain weight right back as soon you replace those lost fluids, but you will rid your body of toxins, and that's a good thing for anyone with diabetes.

My final two body therapies—aromatherapy and music therapy—elevate mood, which is certainly an issue when you're dealing with a serious disease like diabetes. In aromatherapy, essential oils from plants, flowers, and spices can be introduced to your skin and pores either by rubbing them in or by inhaling their aromas. The use of these essential oils will give you an emotional lift if you're struggling with your condition. Try rubbing a few drops of myrtle, coriander, hyssop, galbanum, or frankincense onto the palms, then cup your hands over your mouth and nose and inhale. A deep breath will invigorate the spirit.

So will listening to soft and soothing music that promotes relaxation and healing. I know what I like when it comes to music therapy: contemporary praise and worship music. No matter what works for you, you'll find that listening to uplifting "mood" music is healing.

Rx THE GREAT PHYSICIAN'S Rx FOR DIABETES: CONDITION YOUR BODY WITH EXERCISE AND BODY THERAPIES

- *Make a commitment and an appointment to exercise at least three times a week.*

- *Incorporate five to fifteen minutes of functional fitness into your daily schedule.*

- *Take a brisk walk and see how much better you feel at the end of the day.*

- *Go to sleep earlier, paying close attention to how much sleep you get before midnight. Do your best to get eight hours of sleep nightly. Remember that sleep is the most important nonnutrient you can incorporate to improve your health.*

- *End your next shower by changing the water temperature to cool (or cold) and standing underneath the spray for one minute.*

- *During your next break from work, sit outside in a chair and face the sun. Soak up the rays for ten or fifteen minutes.*

- *Incorporate essential oils into your daily life.*

- *Play worship music in your home, in your car, or on your iPod. Focus on God's plan for your life.*

Take Action

To learn how to incorporate the principles of conditioning your body with exercise and body therapies into your daily regimen, please turn to page 73 for the Great Physician's Rx for Diabetes Battle Plan.

KEY #5

Reduce Toxins in Your Environment

In my last chapter, I introduced Ron Cook, a correctional officer from Wichita, Kansas. There's something more you should know about Ron's story because it relates directly to the topic of this chapter, which is reducing the amount of toxins in your environment.

Ron told me that after reading an earlier book of mine, *Patient, Heal Thyself,* he put two and two together: the reason why his gut was so "messed up," as he described it, was from mercury poisoning in his body, which would come from the foods he ate and amalgam fillings in his teeth. When he adopted the principles behind the *Great Physician's Rx for Health and Wellness,* however, his blood sugar levels were cut in half. But check this out: one time when he went swimming in a heavily chlorinated pool, his blood sugar levels shot back up to their old levels again!

Stories like Ron's remind me that we all have toxins inside our bodies because they are present everywhere in our environment—the air we breathe, the water we drink or swim in, the lotions and cosmetics we rub on our skin, the products we use to clean our homes, and even the toothpaste we dab on our toothbrushes. If your blood and urine were tested, lab technicians would uncover dozens of toxins in your bloodstream, including PCBs (polychlorinated biphenyls), dioxins, furans, trace metals, phthalates, VOCs (volatile organic compounds), and chlorine.

Some toxins are water soluble, meaning they are rapidly passed out of the body and present little harm. Unfortunately many more toxins are fat soluble, meaning that it can take months or years before they are completely eliminated from your system. Some of the better known fat-soluble toxins are dioxins, phthalates, and chlorine, and when they are not eliminated from the body, they become stored in your fatty tissues. "Consider those love handles as a hiding place for stored toxins and poisons," says Don Colbert, M.D. and author of *Toxic Relief.* "In other words, fat is usually toxic, too."[1]

The best way to flush fat-soluble toxins out of your bloodstream is to increase your intake of drinking water (which I'll get into shortly) so that you will excrete toxins via the kidneys and urinary tract; consume a whole food fiber/green food blend to aid in the elimination of toxins from the bowel; increase perspiration through exercise and sauna baths to eliminate toxins through the lymphatic system; and practice deep breathing to eliminate toxins from the lungs. Dietary detoxification strategies include increasing the intake of high-enzyme raw fruits and vegetables, increasing dietary fiber, and eating leaner meats, especially grass-fed or pastured beef or bison and wild-caught fish. Remember: most commercially produced beef, chicken, and pork act as chemical magnets for toxins in the environment, so they will not be as healthy as eating grass-fed beef. In addition, consuming organic produce purchased at health food stores, roadside stands, and farmers' markets will expose you to less pesticide residues, as compared to conventionally grown fruits and vegetables.

Canned tuna, because of its high mercury levels, is another

food to be careful of, which is why I recommend no more than two cans of tuna per week. Due to environmental contamination, metallic particles of mercury, lead, and aluminum continue to be found in the fatty tissues of tuna, swordfish, and king mackerel. Shrimp and lobster, which are shellfish that scavenge the ocean floor, are unclean meats that should be eliminated from your diet.

WHAT TO DRINK

Every diet book on the shelf touts the health benefits of drinking water, and I second that advice. Water is especially important because of its ability to flush out toxins and other metabolic wastes from the body, and overweight people with diabetes tend to have larger metabolic loads.

Increasing your intake of water will speed up your metabolism—which can lead to weight loss—and allow your body to assimilate nutrients from the foods you eat and the nutritional supplements you take. Since water is the primary resource for carrying nutrients throughout the body, a lack of adequate hydration results in metabolic wastes accumulating in your body—a form of self-poisoning. That's why I preach that the importance of drinking enough water cannot be overstated: water is a life force involved in nearly every bodily process, from efficient digestion to healthy blood circulation.

Yet many with diabetes eschew water for a pale imitation—diet drinks, thinking that sodas like Diet Coke, Diet Dr. Pepper, and Diet Pepsi are okay to drink because they do not contain any sugar. I believe, however, that these diet drinks are just as bad or worse for diabetics than regular soda because they contain artificial sweeteners like aspartame, acesulfame K, or sucralose.

Even though the Food and Drug Administration has approved the use of artificial sweeteners in drinks (and foods), these chemical food additives may prove to be detrimental to your health in the long term. And if you're thinking that "energy drinks" like Red Bull and Sobe Adrenaline Rush are a solution to hydration, then let me remind you that these drinks come "fortified" with caffeine and unhealthy amino acids.

Nothing beats plain old water for those with diabetes, especially those who are obese. Diabetics should take note of what F. Batmanghelidj, M.D. and author of *You're Not Sick, You're Thirsty!*, says about the topic:

> Dry mouth is one of the very last indicators of dehydration of the body. By the time dry mouth becomes an indicator of water shortage, many delicate functions of the body have been shut down and prepared for depletion. A dehydrated body loses sophistication and versatility. One example is juvenile diabetes, in which the insulin-producing cells of the pancreas are sacrificed as a result of persistent dehydration.[2]

So for the second time in this book, I urge you to drink a lot of water. Cold or lukewarm, it doesn't matter. Water helps you digest your meals more efficiently, reduces fluid retention, and prevents constipation. You'll also notice a difference in your skin as water reduces the appearance of wrinkles and gives the skin a healthy glow.

I don't recommend drinking water straight from the tap, however. Nearly all municipal water is routinely treated with chlorine, a potent bacteria-killing chemical, as my friend Ron Cook found out. I've installed a whole-house filtration system that removes the chlorine and other impurities from the water *before* it enters our household pipes. Nicki and I can confidently turn on the tap and enjoy the health benefits of chlorine-free water for drinking, cooking, and bathing. Since our water doesn't have a chemical aftertaste, we're more apt to drink it.

A good rule of thumb is that you should drink one quart of water for every fifty pounds of weight, so if you weigh more than 200 pounds, then you should be drinking one full gallon of water daily. I know what you're thinking: *Jordan, if I drink that much water, I can never be farther than fifteen steps from a bathroom.* Yes, you will probably treble your trips to the toilet, but trust me on this: if you're serious about controlling your blood sugar and losing weight, you must be serious about drinking enough water. There's no other physiological way for you to rid yourself of fat reserves and toxins stored inside your body.

TOXINS ELSEWHERE IN YOUR ENVIRONMENT

There are other toxins not directly related to diabetes and obesity but are important enough to mention.

Plastics

Although I occasionally drink bottled waters from plastic containers, I think it's safer to drink water from glass because dioxins and phthalates added in the manufacturing process of plastic can leach into the water, especially after reuse of the same bottle more than once.

Air Quality

We spend 90 percent of our time indoors, usually in well-insulated and energy-efficient homes and offices with central air-conditioning in the summer and forced-air heating during the winter. Double-pane windows, when tamped down shut, don't allow any fresh air into the home, and they trap "used" air filled with harmful particles such as carbon dioxide, nitrogen dioxide, and pet dander.

Perhaps you've noticed all the attention given to mold-related illnesses and homes that have been torn up to rid walls and studs of spores of green and black mold. Those living in mold-infested environments have been diagnosed with impaired thyroid and adrenal problems, chronic fatigue, and memory impairment. It's tough to stick with a lifestyle change—or remember to do so—if poor indoor air quality drains your energy.

I recommend opening your doors and windows periodically to freshen the air you breathe, even if the temperatures are blazing hot or downright freezing. Just a few minutes of fresh air will do wonders.

I also advise the purchase of a quality air filter, which will remove tiny airborne particles of dust, soot, pollen, mold, and dander. I have set up four air purifiers in our home that scrub harmful impurities out of the air.

Household Cleaners

Many of today's commercial household cleaners contain potentially harmful chemicals and solvents that expose people to VOCs—volatile organic compounds—which can cause eye, nose, and throat irritation.

Nicki and I have found that natural ingredients like vinegar, lemon juice, and baking soda are excellent substances that make our home spick-and-span. Natural cleaning products that aren't harsh, abrasive, or potentially dangerous to your family are available in natural food stores.

Skin Care and Body Care Products

Toxic chemicals such as chemical solvents and phthalates are found in lipstick, lip gloss, lip conditioner, hair coloring, hair spray, shampoo, and soap. Ladies, when you rub a tube of lipstick across your lips, your skin readily absorbs these toxins, and that's unhealthy. As with the case regarding household cleaners, you can find natural cosmetics in progressive natural food markets, although they are becoming more widely available in drugstores and beauty stores.

FINAL THOUGHT

In closing, let me be very clear that you most likely will not get sick immediately from drinking chlorinated water, breathing in recirculated air, using commercial household cleaners, rubbing chemical-laden shampoo in your hair, or even brushing your teeth with artificially flavored toothpaste, but the consistent use of these products can erode good health. By the time you notice symptoms, the damage may have already been done.

R℞ THE GREAT PHYSICIAN'S Rx FOR DIABETES: REDUCE TOXINS IN YOUR ENVIRONMENT

- *Drink the minimum recommended amount of eight glasses of water daily.*

- *Use glass containers instead of plastic containers whenever possible.*

- *Improve indoor air quality by opening windows and buying an air filtration system.*

- *Use natural cleaning products for your home.*

- *Use natural products for skin care, body care, hair care, cosmetics, and toothpaste.*

- *Don't smoke cigarettes or use tobacco products.*

Take Action

To learn how to incorporate the principles of reducing
toxins in your environment into your daily regimen,
please turn to page 73 for the Great Physician's Rx for
Diabetes Battle Plan.

KEY #6

Avoid Deadly Emotions

Did you know that anger, acrimony, apprehension, agitation, anxiety, and alarm are deadly emotions, and when you experience any of these feelings—whether justified or not—the efficiency of your immune system decreases noticeably for six hours? (This is the same amount of time your immune system shuts down when you eat large amounts of sugar.)

In addition, depression, stress, and worry may increase the risk of developing type 2 diabetes, according to a recent medical study published in *Diabetes Care*.[1] I believe negative emotions can adversely affect your health and produce lethal toxins that threaten body and spirit. My friend Don Colbert, M.D., author of the fine book *Deadly Emotions* (Thomas Nelson, 2003), says that an emotional roller coaster saps a person of both physical and psychological health, which often leaves body and mind depleted of energy and strength. Dr. Colbert points out that medical studies dealing with unhealthy emotions show that

- the mind and the body are linked, which means how you feel emotionally can determine how you feel physically.

- certain emotions release hormones into the body that can trigger the development of a host of diseases.

- researchers have directly and scientifically linked deadly emotions to hypertension, cardiovascular disease, and diseases related to the immune system.
- those fighting depression have an increased risk of developing cancer, heart disease, and diabetes, as mentioned earlier.

Deadly emotions alter the chemistry of your body, and unchecked emotions can be a pervasive force in determining your daily behavior. Eating while under stress causes the liver's bile tubes to narrow, which blocks bile from reaching the small intestine, where food is waiting to be digested. This is not healthy for those with diabetes. An old proverb states it well: "What you are eating is not nearly as important as what's eating you."

That's wise advice, but it's been my experience that when stress overwhelms people's lives, they tend to fall off the healthy food wagon. When life overwhelms them, they revert to old habits: nibbling on sweets or oily chips, raiding the refrigerator, or ordering in. They hunt down extremely pleasurable foods filled with fat and sugar—Belgian chocolates or Ben & Jerry's Cherry Garcia Ice Cream—to dampen stress and ameliorate symptoms of depression. They eat all the wrong foods to take their minds off their troubles.

These deadly emotions can produce toxins similar to a diabetic bingeing on a dozen glazed doughnuts. Those who are obese often have difficulty forgiving those who teased them about their body shape, made snide comments about their plus-size clothes, or told them that they'll never lose weight.

If you've been hurt in the past by mean-spirited comments, I'm sure I'm not the first person to urge you to put the past in the rearview mirror and move forward. But you must. If you follow my principles for a healthy lifestyle, I'm confident that this will help you deal with any deadly emotions. Please remember that no matter how bad you've been hurt in the past, it's still possible to forgive. "If you forgive men their trespasses, your heavenly Father will also forgive you," Jesus said in Matthew 6. "But if you do not forgive men their trespasses, neither will your Father forgive your trespasses" (vv. 14–15).

Give those who tormented you your forgiveness, and then let it go.

R̹ THE GREAT PHYSICIAN'S Rx FOR DIABETES: AVOID DEADLY EMOTIONS

- *Don't eat when you're sad, scared, or stressed by everyday life.*

- *Recognize the interaction between having deadly emotions and having diabetes.*

- *Trust God when you face circumstances that cause you to worry or become anxious.*

- *Practice forgiveness every day and forgive those who hurt you.*

Take Action

To learn how to incorporate the principles of avoiding deadly emotions into your daily regimen, please turn to page 73 for the Great Physician's Rx for Diabetes Battle Plan.

KEY #7

Live a Life of Prayer and Purpose

Prayer is the foundation of a healthy life, linking your body, soul, and spirit to God. Prayer is a two-way communication with our Creator, the God of the universe. There's power in prayer: "The prayer of faith will save the sick" (James 5:15).

Prayer is the way we talk to God. There is no greater source of power than talking to the One who made us. Prayer is not a formality. Prayer is not about religion. Prayer is about a relationship—the hotline to heaven. We can talk to God anytime, anywhere, for any reason. He is always there to listen, and He always has our best interests at heart because we are His children.

If you decide to adopt the principles behind *The Great Physician's Rx for Diabetes* for your life, I urge you to undergird your effort with prayer, which will give you the perseverance to prevail against this disease. Seal all that you do with the power of prayer, and watch your life become more than you ever thought possible.

I'm not guaranteeing that you will experience a miraculous cure or that astonishing things will happen to you, although they often do. But I will tell you that if you treat your body as God meant for you to treat it—like a temple of the Holy Spirit (1 Cor. 6:19–20)—God will honor that.

You know, heavyset people with diabetes often ask me if overeating is a sin. While the Bible has little direct criticism of gluttony, the book of Proverbs describes the social and economic disadvantages of gluttony, which is defined as excess in eating and drinking: "Do not mix with winebibbers, or with gluttonous eaters of meat; for the drunkard and the glutton will come to poverty, and drowsiness will clothe a man with rags," says Proverbs 23:20–21.

Here's where I come down on the topic. If you're wondering whether you can overeat and not deal with the root causes of your diabetes and still get to heaven, my response is yes, you'll get to heaven. You'll just get there a lot sooner.

When you follow God's health plan, however, you'll honor your family, and the best way to honor them is by staying here on earth. I always cringe when I hear about someone involved in ministry—the pastorate, the mission field, vacation Bible school—who dies way too early because he or she did not take care of his or her body. That's a waste of God's resources here on earth.

God has a purpose for your life, and when you're called to serve Him in ministry, as I believe all of us are, every minute is precious. Every year we have more to offer, not less, because we have wisdom and experience on our side. Use that wisdom by establishing a health legacy for your future generations, and you won't live a life of regrets.

You may be reading this and thinking, *I know my diabetes is a ticking time bomb . . . and I'm not sure what my future holds.* Well, you've been given the knowledge to do something about your disease from this day forward. My question to you is: How are you going to act upon what you've learned from *The Great Physician's Rx for Diabetes?*

It matters, you know. Both of my father's grandparents had diabetes, and my mother's grandmother, Gramma Simma, had a gangrenous leg amputated late in life, which everyone in our family assumes was caused by undiagnosed diabetes.

On my father's side, my great-grandmother, Lena, died in the late 1960s because of complications of diabetes. She was very sick in her later years, suffering several strokes because her doctors couldn't get her diabetes under control. Her husband, my great-grandfather, Jacob, was also diabetic all his life, which turned out to be a long one. He died at the age of eighty-eight, but my father, who loved his grandfather very much, says he left before his time. "Poppy," he said, "wasn't insulin dependent, but he had to take medication. The night he died, he suffered a heart attack, and a pen or something in his pajama pocket punctured his heart, and he died instantly. This tragic event happened two days after my wife's father died."

As for myself, I haven't forgotten the memory of my grandfather on my father's side, who was significantly overweight, passing away at the age of sixty-two from a heart attack. My grandfather on my mother's side was overweight as well, and he died of a heart attack at the age of sixty-five. Both of my grandfathers were gone before I turned ten years old.

You don't have to die early from complications of diabetes. Give yourself the best chance to be there for your loved ones by following the principles behind *The Great Physician's Rx for Diabetes*.

Now it's your turn to take the first step on your new road to wellness. Welcome to your new, healthy life!

Start a Small Group

It's difficult to face a health challenge alone. If you have friends or family members struggling with diabetes or other health problems, or if you know people who just want to live the healthy life God intended, ask them to join you in following the Great Physician's prescription for better health. You can learn how to become a small group leader in your community or find an existing small group in your area by visiting www.GreatPhysiciansRx.com.

R THE GREAT PHYSICIAN'S Rx FOR DIABETES: LIVE A LIFE OF PRAYER AND PURPOSE

- *Pray continually.*

- *Confess God's promises upon waking and before you retire.*

- *Find God's purpose for your life and live it every day.*

- *Be an agent of change in your life. Only you can take that first step toward reversing diabetes in your life.*

Take Action

To learn how to incorporate the principles of living a
life of prayer and purpose into your daily regimen,
please turn to page 73 for the Great Physician's Rx for
Diabetes Battle Plan.

THE GREAT PHYSICIAN'S RX
FOR DIABETES BATTLE PLAN

Upon Waking

Prayer: thank God because this is the day that the Lord has made. Rejoice and be glad in it. Thank Him for the breath in your lungs and the life in your body. Ask the Lord to heal your body and use your experience to benefit the lives of others. Read Matthew 6:9–13 out loud.

Purpose: ask the Lord to give you an opportunity to add significance to someone's life today. Watch for that opportunity. Ask God to use you this day for His intended purpose.

Advanced hygiene: for hands and nails, jab fingers into semisoft soap four or five times, and lather hands with soap for fifteen seconds, rubbing soap over cuticles and rinsing under water as warm as you can stand. Take another swab of semisoft soap into your hands and wash your face. Next, fill basin or sink with water as warm as you can stand, and add one to three tablespoons of table salt and one to three eye-droppers of iodine-based mineral solution. Dunk face into water and open eyes, blinking repeatedly underwater. Keep eyes open underwater for three seconds. After cleaning your eyes, put your face back in the water, and close your mouth while blowing bubbles out of your nose. Come up from the water, and immerse your face in the water once again, gently taking water into your nostrils and expelling bubbles. Come up from the water, and blow your nose into facial tissue. To cleanse the ears, use hydrogen peroxide and mineral-based ear drops, putting two or three drops into each ear and letting stand for sixty seconds. Tilt your head to expel the drops. For the teeth, apply two or three drops of essential oil-based tooth drops to the toothbrush. This can be used to brush your teeth or added to existing toothpaste. After brushing your teeth, brush your tongue for fifteen seconds. (Visit www.BiblicalHealthInstitute.com and click on the GPRx Resource Guide for recommended advanced hygiene products.)

Reduce toxins: open windows for one hour today. Use natural soap and natural skin and body care products (shower gel, body creams, etc.). Use natural facial care products. Use natural toothpaste. Use natural hair care products such as shampoo, conditioner, gel, mousse, and hairspray. (Visit www.BiblicalHealthInstitute.com and click on the GPRx Resource Guide for recommended products.)

Supplements: take one serving of a fiber/green superfood powder (mixed) or five caplets of a super green formula swallowed with twelve to sixteen ounces of water. (For recommended products, visit www.BiblicalHealthInstitute.com and click on the GPRx Resource Guide.)

Body therapy: get twenty minutes of direct sunlight sometime during the day, but be careful between the hours of 10:00 a.m. and 2:00 p.m.

Exercise: perform functional fitness exercises for five to fifteen minutes, or spend five to fifteen minutes on a mini trampoline. Finish with five to ten minutes of deep-breathing exercises. (One to three rounds of the exercises can be found at www.GreatPhysiciansRx.com.)

Emotional health: whenever you face a circumstance, such as your health, that causes you to worry, repeat the following: "Lord, I trust You. I cast my cares upon You, and I believe that You're going to take care of [insert your current situation] and make my health and make my body strong." Confess that throughout the day whenever you think about your health condition.

Breakfast

Make a vanilla-cinnamon smoothie in a blender with the following ingredients:

one cup plain whole milk yogurt or kefir (goat's milk is best); one tablespoon organic flaxseed oil; one tablespoon organic raw honey; one-half fresh or frozen organic banana; two tablespoons goat's milk protein powder (for recommended products, visit www.BiblicalHealthInstitute.com and click on the GPRx Resource Guide); one-fourth teaspoon organic ground cinnamon; dash of vanilla extract

Supplements: take two whole food multivitamin caplets and one capsule of a whole food antioxidant/energy formula with B vitamins, folic acid, and chromium (for recommended products, visit www.BiblicalHealthInstitute.com and click on the GPRx Resource Guide).

Lunch

Before eating, drink eight ounces of water.

During lunch, drink cinnamon green chai hot tea (for recommended products, visit www.BiblicalHealthInstitute.com and click on the GPRx Resource Guide) with one teaspoon of raw honey.

large green salad with mixed greens, avocado, carrots, cucumbers, celery, tomatoes, red cabbage, red peppers, red onions, and sprouts with three hard-boiled omega-3 eggs

salad dressing: use extra virgin olive oil, apple cider vinegar or lemon juice, Celtic sea salt, herbs, and spices, or mix one tablespoon of extra virgin olive oil with one tablespoon of a healthy store-bought dressing

two ounces of applesauce with one-fourth teaspoon of organic ground cinnamon

Supplements: take two whole food multivitamin caplets and one capsule of a whole food antioxidant/energy formula with B vitamins, folic acid, and chromium.

Dinner

Before eating, drink eight ounces of water.

During dinner, drink cinnamon green chai hot tea with one teaspoon of raw honey.

baked, poached, or grilled wild-caught salmon

steamed broccoli

large green salad with mixed greens, avocado, carrots, cucumbers, celery, tomatoes, red cabbage, red onions, red peppers, and sprouts

salad dressing: use extra virgin olive oil, apple cider vinegar or lemon juice, Celtic ea salt, herbs, and spices, or mix one tablespoon of extra virgin olive oil with one tablespoon of a healthy store-bought dressing

Supplements: take two whole food multivitamin caplets and one capsule of a whole food antioxidant/energy formula with B vitamins, folic acid, and chromium and one to three teaspoons or three to nine capsules of a high omega-3 cod liver oil complex (for recommended products, visit www.BiblicalHealthInstitute.com and click on the GPRx Resource Guide).

Snacks

apple slices with raw sesame butter (tahini)

one whole food nutrition bar with beta-glucans from soluble oat fiber (for recommended products, visit www.BiblicalHealthInstitute.com and click on the GPRx Resource Guide)

Drink eight to twelve ounces of water.

Before Bed

Exercise: go for a walk outdoors or participate in a favorite sport or recreational activity.

Supplements: take one serving of a fiber/green superfood powder (mixed) or five caplets of a super green formula swallowed with twelve to sixteen ounces of water.

Body therapy: take a warm bath for fifteen minutes with eight drops of biblical essential oils added.

Advanced hygiene: repeat the advanced hygiene instructions from the morning of Day 1.

Emotional health: ask the Lord to bring to your mind someone you need to forgive. Take out a sheet of paper and write the person's name at the top. Try to remember each specific action that person did against you that brought you pain. Write down the following: "I forgive [insert person's name] for [insert the action he or she did against you]." After you fill up the paper, tear it up or burn it, and ask God to give you the strength to truly forgive that person.

Purpose: ask yourself these questions: "Did I live a life of purpose today?" "What did I do to add value to someone else's life today?" Commit to living a day of purpose tomorrow.

Prayer: thank God for this day, asking Him to give you a restoring night's rest and a fresh start tomorrow. Thank Him for His steadfast love that never ceases and His mercies that are new every morning. Read Romans 8:35, 37–39 out loud.

Sleep: go to bed by 10:30 p.m.

Day 2

Upon Waking

Prayer: thank God because this is the day that the Lord has made. Rejoice and be glad in it. Thank Him for the breath in your lungs and the life in your body. Ask the Lord to heal your body and use your experience to benefit the lives of others. Read Psalm 91 out loud.

Purpose: ask the Lord to give you an opportunity to add significance to someone's life today. Watch for that opportunity. Ask God to use you this day for His intended purpose.

Advanced hygiene: follow the advanced hygiene recommendations from the morning of Day 1.

Reduce toxins: follow the recommendations to reduce toxins from the morning of Day 1.

Supplements: take one serving of a fiber/green superfood powder (mixed) or five caplets of a super green formula swallowed with twelve to sixteen ounces of water.

Body therapy: take a hot and cold shower. After a normal shower, alternate sixty seconds of water as hot as you can stand it, followed by sixty seconds of water as cold as you can stand it. Repeat cycle four times for a total of eight minutes, finishing with cold.

Exercise: perform functional fitness exercises for five to fifteen minutes or spend five to fifteen minutes on a mini trampoline. Finish with five to ten minutes of deep-breathing exercises. (One to three rounds of the exercises can be found at www.GreatPhysiciansRx.com.)

Emotional health: follow the emotional health recommendations from the morning of Day 1.

Breakfast

two or three eggs any style, cooked in one tablespoon of extra virgin coconut oil (for recommended products, visit www.BiblicalHealthInstitute.com and click on the GPRx Resource Guide)

one slice of cinnamon-raisin sprouted or yeast-free whole grain bread (for recommended products, visit www.BiblicalHealthInstitute.com and click on the GPRx Resource Guide) with one-fourth teaspoon cinnamon, butter, and honey

one cup of spicy black chai hot tea with one teaspoon of raw honey

Supplements: take two whole food multivitamin caplets and one capsule of a whole food antioxidant/energy formula with B vitamins, folic acid, and chromium.

Lunch

Before eating, drink eight ounces of water.

During lunch, drink spicy black chai hot tea with one teaspoon of raw honey.

large green salad with mixed greens, avocado, carrots, tomatoes, red cabbage, red onions, red peppers, and sprouts with three ounces of cold, poached, or canned wild salmon

salad dressing: use extra virgin olive oil, apple cider vinegar or lemon juice, Celtic sea salt, herbs, and spices, or mix one tablespoon of extra virgin olive oil with one tablespoon of a healthy store-bought dressing

two ounces of organic applesauce mixed with one-fourth teaspoon of organic ground cinnamon

Supplements: take two whole food multivitamin caplets and one capsule of a whole food antioxidant/energy formula with B vitamins, folic acid, and chromium.

Dinner

Before eating, drink eight ounces of water.

During dinner, drink spicy black chai hot tea with one teaspoon of raw honey.

roasted organic chicken

cooked vegetables (carrots, onions, or peas, etc.)

large green salad with mixed greens, avocado, carrots, tomatoes, red cabbage, red onions, red peppers, and sprouts salad dressing: use extra virgin olive oil, apple cider vinegar or lemon juice, Celtic sea salt, herbs, and spices, or mix one tablespoon of extra virgin olive oil with one tablespoon of a healthy store-bought dressing

Supplements: take two whole food multivitamin caplets and one capsule of a whole food antioxidant/energy formula with B vitamins, folic acid, and chromium and one to three teaspoons or three to nine capsules of a high omega-3 cod-liver oil complex.

Snacks

three ounces of cottage cheese mixed with one tablespoon of flaxseed oil, one teaspoon of organic raw honey, and one-fourth teaspoon of organic ground cinnamon

one whole food nutrition bar with beta-glucans from soluble oat fiber

Drink eight to twelve ounces of water, or hot or iced fresh-brewed tea with honey.

Before Bed

Exercise: go for a walk outdoors or participate in a favorite sport or recreational activity.

Supplements: take one serving of a fiber/green superfood powder (mixed) or five caplets of a super green formula swallowed with twelve to sixteen ounces of water.

Advanced hygiene: repeat the advanced hygiene instructions from the morning of Day 1.

Emotional health: repeat the emotional health recommendations from the evening of Day 1.

Purpose: ask yourself these questions: "Did I live a life of purpose today?" "What did I do to add value to someone else's life today?" Commit to living a day of purpose tomorrow.

Prayer: thank God for this day, asking Him to give you a restoring night's rest and a fresh start tomorrow. Thank Him for His steadfast love that never ceases and His mercies there are new every morning. Read 1 Corinthians 13:4–8 out loud.

Body therapy: spend ten minutes listening to soothing music before you retire.

Sleep: go to bed by 10:30 p.m.

DAY 3

Upon Waking

Prayer: thank God because this is the day that the Lord has made. Rejoice and be glad in it. Thank Him for the breath in your lungs and the life in your body. Ask the Lord to heal your body and use your experience to benefit the lives of others. Read Ephesians 6:13–18 out loud.

Purpose: ask the Lord to give you an opportunity to add significance to someone's life today. Watch for that opportunity. Ask God to use you this day for His intended purpose.

Advanced hygiene: follow the advanced hygiene recommendations from the morning of Day 1.

Reduce toxins: follow the recommendations to reduce toxins from the morning of Day 1.

Supplements: take one serving of a fiber/green superfood powder (mixed) or five caplets of a super green formula swallowed with twelve to sixteen ounces of water.

Body therapy: get twenty minutes of direct sunlight sometime during the day, but be careful between the hours of 10:00 a.m. and 2:00 p.m.

Exercise: perform functional fitness exercises for five to fifteen minutes or spend five to fifteen minutes on a mini trampoline. Finish with five to ten minutes of deep-breathing exercises. (One to three rounds of the exercises can be found at www.GreatPhysiciansRx.com.)

Emotional health: follow the emotional health recommendations from the morning of Day 1.

Breakfast

four to eight ounces of organic whole milk yogurt or cottage cheese with fruit (pineapple, peaches, or berries), honey, one-fourth teaspoon of organic ground cinnamon, and a dash of vanilla extract

handful of raw almonds

one cup of cinnamon green chai hot tea with one teaspoon of raw honey

Supplements: take two whole food multivitamin caplets and one capsule of a whole food antioxidant/energy formula with B vitamins, folic acid, and chromium.

Lunch

Before eating, drink eight ounces of water.

During lunch, drink cinnamon green chai hot tea with one teaspoon of raw honey.

large green salad with mixed greens, avocado, carrots, cucumbers, celery, tomatoes, red cabbage, red peppers, red onions, and sprouts with two ounces of low mercury, high omega-3 canned tuna (for recommended products, visit www.BiblicalHealthInstitute.com and click on the GPRx Resource Guide)

salad dressing: use extra virgin olive oil, apple cider vinegar or lemon juice, Celtic sea salt, herbs, and spices, or mix one tablespoon of extra virgin olive oil with one tablespoon of a healthy store-bought dressing

one piece of fruit in season

Supplements: take two whole food multivitamin caplets and one capsule of a whole food antioxidant/energy formula with B vitamins, folic acid, and chromium.

Dinner

Before eating, drink eight ounces of water.

During dinner, drink cinnamon green chai hot tea with one teaspoon of raw honey.

red meat steak (beef, buffalo, or venison)

steamed broccoli

baked sweet potato with butter

large green salad with mixed greens, avocado, carrots, cucumbers, celery, tomatoes, red cabbage, red peppers, red onions, and sprouts

salad dressing: use extra virgin olive oil, apple cider vinegar or lemon juice, Celtic sea salt, herbs, and spices, or mix one tablespoon of extra virgin olive oil with one tablespoon of a healthy store-bought dressing

Supplements: take two whole food multivitamin caplets and one capsule of a whole food antioxidant/energy formula with B vitamins, folic acid, and chromium and one to three teaspoons or three to nine capsules of a high omega-3 cod-liver oil complex.

Snacks

four ounces of cottage cheese or whole milk yogurt with one-fourth teaspoon organic ground cinnamon, organic raw honey, and a few almonds and raisins

one whole food nutrition bar with beta-glucans from soluble oat fiber

Drink eight to twelve ounces of water, or hot or iced fresh-brewed tea with honey.

Before Bed

Exercise: go for a walk outdoors or participate in a favorite sport or recreational activity.

Supplements: take one serving of a fiber/green superfood powder (mixed) or five caplets of a super green formula swallowed with twelve to sixteen ounces of water.

Body therapy: take a warm bath for fifteen minutes with eight drops of biblical essential oils added.

Advanced hygiene: follow the advanced hygiene instructions from the morning of Day 1.

Emotional health: follow the forgiveness recommendations from the evening of Day 1.

Purpose: ask yourself these questions: "Did I live a life of purpose today?" "What did I do to add value to someone else's life today?" Commit to living a day of purpose tomorrow.

Prayer: thank God for this day, asking Him to give you a restoring night's rest and a fresh start tomorrow. Thank Him for His steadfast love that never ceases and His mercies that are new every morning. Read Philippians 4:4–8, 11–13, 19 out loud.

Sleep: go to bed by 10:30 p.m.

Day 4

Upon Waking

Prayer: thank God because this is the day that the Lord has made. Rejoice and be glad in it. Thank Him for the breath in your lungs and the life in your body. Read Matthew 6:9–13 out loud.

Purpose: ask the Lord to give you an opportunity to add significance to someone's life today. Watch for that opportunity. Ask God to use you this day for His intended purpose.

Advanced hygiene: follow the advanced hygiene recommendations from the morning of Day 1.

Reduce toxins: follow the recommendations for reducing toxins from the morning of Day 1.

Supplements: take one serving of a fiber/green superfood powder (mixed) or five caplets of a super green formula swallowed with twelve to sixteen ounces of water.

Exercise: perform functional fitness exercises for five to fifteen minutes or spend five to fifteen minutes on a mini trampoline. Finish with five to ten minutes of deep-breathing exercises. (One to three rounds of the exercises can be found at www.GreatPhysiciansRx.com.)

Body therapy: take a hot and cold shower. After a normal shower, alternate sixty seconds of water as hot as you can stand it, followed by sixty seconds of water as cold as you can stand it. Repeat cycle four times for a total of eight minutes, finishing with cold.

Emotional health: follow the emotional health recommendations from the morning of Day 1.

Breakfast

three soft-boiled or poached eggs

four ounces of sprouted whole grain cereal with two ounces of whole milk yogurt, one-fourth teaspoon organic ground cinnamon, almonds, and raisins (for recommended products, visit www.BiblicalHealthInstitute.com and click on the GPRx Resource Guide)

one cup of spicy black chai hot tea with one teaspoon of raw honey

Supplements: take two whole food multivitamin caplets and one capsule of a whole food antioxidant/energy formula with B vitamins, folic acid, and chromium.

Lunch

Before eating, drink eight ounces of water.

During lunch, drink spicy black chai hot tea with one teaspoon of raw honey.

large green salad with mixed greens, avocado, carrots, cucumbers, celery, tomatoes, red cabbage, red peppers, red onions, and sprouts with two ounces of low mercury, high omega-3 canned tuna

salad dressing: use extra virgin olive oil, apple cider vinegar or lemon juice, Celtic sea salt, herbs, and spices, or mix one tablespoon of extra virgin olive oil with one tablespoon of a healthy store-bought dressing

two ounces of organic applesauce with one-fourth teaspoon of organic ground cinnamon

Supplements: take two whole food multivitamin caplets and one capsule of a whole food antioxidant/energy formula with B vitamins, folic acid, and chromium.

Dinner

Before eating, drink eight ounces of water.

During dinner, drink spicy black chai hot tea with one teaspoon of raw honey.

grilled chicken breast

steamed veggies

small portion of cooked whole grain (quinoa, amaranth, millet, or brown rice) cooked with one tablespoon of extra virgin coconut oil

large green salad with mixed greens, avocado, carrots, cucumbers, celery, tomatoes, red cabbage, red peppers, red onions, and sprouts

salad dressing: use extra virgin olive oil, apple cider vinegar or lemon juice, Celtic sea salt, herbs, and spices, or mix one tablespoon of extra virgin olive oil with one tablespoon of a healthy store-bought dressing

Supplements: take two whole food multivitamin caplets and one capsule of a whole food antioxidant/energy formula with B vitamins, folic acid, and chromium and one to three teaspoons or three to nine capsules of a high omega-3 cod-liver oil complex.

Snacks

apple and carrots with raw almond butter

one whole food nutrition bar with beta-glucans from soluble oat fiber

Drink eight to twelve ounces of water, or hot or iced fresh-brewed tea with honey.

Before Bed

Drink eight to twelve ounces of water or hot tea with honey.

Exercise: go for a walk outdoors or participate in a favorite sport or recreational activity.

Supplements: take one serving of a fiber/green superfood powder (mixed) or five caplets of a super green formula swallowed with twelve to sixteen ounces of water.

Advanced hygiene: follow the advanced hygiene recommendations from the morning of Day 1.

Emotional health: follow the forgiveness recommendations from the evening of Day 1.

Purpose: ask yourself these questions: "Did I live a life of purpose today?" "What did I do to add value to someone else's life today?" Commit to living a day of purpose tomorrow.

Prayer: thank God for this day, asking Him to give you a restoring night's rest and a fresh start tomorrow. Thank Him for His steadfast love that never ceases and His mercies that are new every morning. Read Romans 8:35, 37–39 out loud.

Body therapy: spend ten minutes listening to soothing music before you retire.

Sleep: go to bed by 10:30 p.m.

DAY 5

Upon Waking

Prayer: thank God because this is the day that the Lord has made. Rejoice and be glad in it. Thank Him for the breath in your lungs and the life in your body. Read Psalm 1 out loud.

Purpose: ask the Lord to give you an opportunity to add significance to someone's life today. Watch for that opportunity. Ask God to use you this day for His intended purpose.

Advanced hygiene: follow the advanced hygiene recommendations from the morning of Day 1.

Reduce toxins: follow the recommendations for reducing toxins from the morning of Day 1.

Supplements: take one serving of a fiber/green superfood powder (mixed) or five caplets of a super green formula swallowed with twelve to sixteen ounces of water.

Exercise: perform functional fitness exercises for five to fifteen minutes or spend five to fifteen minutes on a mini trampoline. Finish with five to ten minutes of deep-breathing exercises.

Body therapy: get twenty minutes of direct sunlight sometime during the day, but be careful between the hours of 10:00 a.m. and 2:00 p.m.

Emotional health: follow the emotional health recommendations from the morning of Day 1.

Breakfast

three fried eggs in one teaspoon of extra virgin coconut oil

one serving of slow-cooked organic oatmeal with one-fourth teaspoon of cinnamon, butter, honey, and raisins

one cup of cinnamon green chai hot tea with one teaspoon of raw honey

Supplements: take two whole food multivitamin caplets and one capsule of a whole food antioxidant/energy formula with B vitamins, folic acid, and chromium.

Lunch

Before eating, drink eight ounces of water.

turkey sandwich on sprouted or yeast-free whole grain bread with natural mayonnaise, mustard, raw cheese, lettuce, and tomato

two ounces of organic applesauce with one-fourth teaspoon of organic ground cinnamon

During lunch, drink cinnamon green chai hot tea with one teaspoon of raw honey.

Supplements: take two whole food multivitamin caplets and one capsule of a whole food antioxidant/energy formula with B vitamins, folic acid, and chromium.

Dinner

Before eating, drink eight ounces of water.

During dinner, drink cinnamon green chai hot tea with one teaspoon of raw honey.

Chicken Soup (visit www.GreatPhysiciansRx.com for recipe)

cultured vegetables (for recommended products, visit www.BiblicalHealthInstitute.com and click on the GPRx Resource Guide)

large green salad with mixed greens, avocado, carrots, cucumbers, celery, tomatoes, red cabbage, red peppers, red onions, and sprouts

salad dressing: use extra virgin olive oil, apple cider vinegar or lemon juice, Celtic sea salt, herbs, and spices, or mix one tablespoon of extra virgin olive oil with one tablespoon of a healthy store-bought dressing

Supplements: take two whole food multivitamin caplets and one capsule of a whole food antioxidant/energy formula with B vitamins, folic acid, and chromium and one to three teaspoons or three to nine capsules of a high omega-3 cod-liver oil complex.

Snacks

One whole food nutrition bar with beta-glucans from soluble oat fiber

one-half cup of blueberries and a handful of almonds

Drink eight to twelve ounces of water.

Before Bed

Drink eight to twelve ounces of water or hot tea with honey.

Exercise: go for a walk outdoors or participate in a favorite sport or recreational activity.

Supplements: take one serving of a fiber/green superfood powder (mixed) or five caplets of a super green formula swallowed with twelve to sixteen ounces of water.

Advanced hygiene: follow the advanced hygiene recommendations from the morning of Day 1.

Emotional health: follow the forgiveness recommendations from the evening of Day 1.

Body therapy: take a warm bath for fifteen minutes with eight drops of biblical essential oils added.

Purpose: ask yourself these questions: "Did I live a life of purpose today?" "What did I do to add value to someone else's life today?" Commit to living a day of purpose tomorrow.

Prayer: thank God for this day, asking Him to give you a restoring night's rest and a fresh start tomorrow. Thank Him for His steadfast love that never ceases and His mercies that are new every morning. Read Matthew 6:25–34 out loud.

Sleep: go to bed by 10:30 p.m.

DAY 6 (REST DAY)

Upon Waking

Prayer: thank God because this is the day that the Lord has made. Rejoice and be glad in it. Thank Him for the breath in your lungs and the life in your body. Read Psalm 23 out loud.

Purpose: ask the Lord to give you an opportunity to add significance to someone's life today. Watch for that opportunity. Ask God to use you this day for His intended purpose.

Advanced hygiene: follow the advanced hygiene recommendations from the morning of Day 1.

Reduce toxins: follow the recommendations for reducing toxins from the morning of Day 1.

Supplements: take one serving of a fiber/green superfood powder (mixed) or five caplets of a super green formula swallowed with twelve to sixteen ounces of water.

Exercise: do no formal exercise since it's a rest day.

Body therapies: do none since it's a rest day.

Emotional health: follow the emotional health recommendations from the morning of Day 1.

Breakfast

two or three eggs cooked any style in one teaspoon of extra virgin coconut oil

one grapefruit

handful of almonds

one cup of cinnamon green chai hot tea with one teaspoon of raw honey

Supplements: take two whole food multivitamin caplets and one capsule of a whole food antioxidant/energy formula with B vitamins, folic acid, and chromium.

Lunch

Before eating, drink eight ounces of water.

During lunch, drink cinnamon green chai hot tea with one teaspoon of raw honey.

large green salad with mixed greens, avocado, carrots, cucumbers, celery, tomatoes, red cabbage, red peppers, red onions, and sprouts with three hard-boiled omega-3 eggs

salad dressing: use extra virgin olive oil, apple cider vinegar or lemon juice, Celtic sea salt, herbs, and spices, or mix one tablespoon of extra virgin olive oil with one tablespoon of a healthy store-bought dressing

two ounces of organic applesauce with one-fourth teaspoon organic ground cinnamon

Supplements: take two whole food multivitamin caplets and one capsule of a whole food antioxidant/energy formula with B vitamins, folic acid, and chromium.

Dinner

Before eating, drink eight ounces of water.

During dinner, drink cinnamon green chai hot tea with one teaspoon of raw honey.

roasted organic chicken

cooked vegetables (carrots, onions, peas, etc.)

large green salad with mixed greens, carrots, cucumbers, celery, tomatoes, red cabbage, red peppers, red onions, and sprouts

salad dressing: use extra virgin olive oil, apple cider vinegar or lemon juice, Celtic sea salt, herbs, and spices, or mix one tablespoon of extra virgin olive oil with one tablespoon of a healthy store-bought dressing

Supplements: take two whole food multivitamin caplets and one capsule of a whole food antioxidant/energy formula with B vitamins, folic acid, and chromium and one to three teaspoons or three to nine capsules of a high omega-3 cod-liver oil complex.

Snacks

handful of raw almonds with apple wedges

one whole food nutrition bar with beta-glucans from soluble oat fiber

Drink eight to twelve ounces of water, or hot or iced fresh-brewed tea with honey.

Before Bed

Drink eight to twelve ounces of water or hot tea with honey.

Exercise: go for a walk outdoors or participate in a favorite sport or recreational activity.

Supplements: take one serving of a fiber/green superfood powder (mixed) or five caplets of a super green formula swallowed with twelve to sixteen ounces of high-alkaline water or raw vegetable juice.

Advanced hygiene: follow the advanced hygiene recommendations from the morning of Day 1.

Emotional health: follow the forgiveness recommendations from the evening of Day 1.

Purpose: ask yourself these questions: "Did I live a life of purpose today?" "What did I do to add value to someone else's life today?" Commit to living a day of purpose tomorrow.

Prayer: thank God for this day, asking Him to give you a restoring night's rest and a fresh start tomorrow. Thank Him for His steadfast love that never ceases and His mercies that are new every morning. Read Psalm 23 out loud.

Body therapy: spend ten minutes listening to soothing music before you retire.

Sleep: go to bed by 10:30 p.m.

DAY 7

Upon Waking

Prayer: thank God because this is the day that the Lord has made. Rejoice and be glad in it. Thank Him for the breath in your lungs and the life in your body. Read Psalm 91 out loud.

Purpose: ask the Lord to give you an opportunity to add significance to someone's life today. Watch for that opportunity. Ask God to use you this day for His intended purpose.

Advanced hygiene: follow the advanced hygiene recommendations from the morning of Day 1.

Reduce toxins: follow the recommendations for reducing toxins from the morning of Day 1.

Supplements: take one serving of a fiber/green superfood powder (mixed) or five caplets of a super green formula swallowed with twelve to sixteen ounces of water.

Exercise: perform functional fitness exercises for five to fifteen minutes or spend five to fifteen minutes on a mini trampoline. Finish with five to ten minutes of deep-breathing exercises.

Body therapy: get twenty minutes of direct sunlight sometime during the day, but be careful between the hours of 10:00 a.m. and 2:00 p.m.

Emotional health: follow the emotional health recommendations from the morning of Day 1.

Breakfast

Make a vanilla-cinnamon smoothie in a blender with the following ingredients:

one cup plain whole milk yogurt or kefir (goat's milk is best)

one tablespoon organic flaxseed oil

one tablespoon organic raw honey

one-half fresh or frozen organic banana

two tablespoons goat's milk protein powder (for recommendations, visit www.BiblicalHealthInstitute.com and click on the GPRx Resource Guide)

one-fourth teaspoon organic ground cinnamon

dash of vanilla extract

Supplements: take two whole food multivitamin caplets and one capsule of a whole food antioxidant/energy formula with B vitamins, folic acid, and chromium.

Lunch

Before eating, drink eight ounces of water.

During lunch, drink cinnamon green chai hot tea with raw honey.

large green salad with mixed greens, raw goat cheese, avocado, carrots, cucumbers, celery, tomatoes, red cabbage, red peppers, red onions, and sprouts with three ounces of cold, poached, or canned wild-caught salmon

salad dressing: use extra virgin olive oil, apple cider vinegar or lemon juice, Celtic sea salt, herbs, and spices, or mix one tablespoon of extra virgin olive oil with one tablespoon of a healthy store-bought dressing

one piece of fruit in season

Supplements: take two whole food multivitamin caplets and one capsule of a whole food antioxidant/energy formula with B vitamins, folic acid, and chromium.

Dinner

Before eating, drink eight ounces of water.

During dinner, drink cinnamon green chai hot tea with raw honey.

baked or grilled fish of your choice

steamed broccoli

baked sweet potato with butter

large green salad with mixed greens, carrots, cucumbers, celery, tomatoes, red cabbage, red peppers, red onions, and sprouts

salad dressing: use extra virgin olive oil, apple cider vinegar or lemon juice, Celtic sea salt, herbs, and spices, or mix one tablespoon of extra virgin olive oil with one tablespoon of a healthy store-bought dressing

Supplements: take two whole food multivitamin caplets and one capsule of a whole food antioxidant/energy formula with B vitamins, folic acid, and chromium and one to three teaspoons or three to nine capsules of a high omega-3 cod-liver oil complex.

Snacks

apple slices with raw sesame butter (tahini)

one whole food nutrition bar with beta-glucans from soluble oat fiber

Drink eight to twelve ounces of water, or hot or iced fresh-brewed tea with honey.

Before Bed

Drink eight to twelve ounces of water or hot tea with honey.

Exercise: go for a walk outdoors or participate in a favorite sport or recreational activity.

Supplements: take one serving of a fiber/green superfood powder (mixed) or five caplets of a super green formula swallowed with twelve to sixteen ounces of high-alkaline water or raw vegetable juice.

Advanced hygiene: follow the advanced hygiene recommendations from the morning of Day 1.

Emotional health: follow the forgiveness recommendations from the evening of Day 1.

Body therapy: take a warm bath for fifteen minutes with eight drops of biblical essential oils added.

Purpose: ask yourself these questions: "Did I live a life of purpose today?" "What did I do to add value to someone else's life today?" Commit to living a day of purpose tomorrow.

Prayer: thank God for this day, asking Him to give you a restoring night's rest and a fresh start tomorrow. Thank Him for His steadfast love that never ceases and His mercies that are new every morning. Read 1 Corinthians 13:4–8 out loud.

Sleep: go to bed by 10:30 p.m.

DAY 8 AND BEYOND

If you are beginning to get better control of your blood sugar and feel better, but still have a way to go on your road to wellness, you can repeat the Great Physician's Rx for Diabetes Battle Plan as many times as you'd like. For detailed step-by-step suggestions and meal and lifestyle plans, visit www.GreatPhysiciansRx.com and join the 40-Day Health Experience (if you want to continue on a strict phase of the health plan) or the Lifetime of Wellness plan (if you want to maintain your newfound level of health). These online programs will provide you with customized daily meal and exercise plans and provide you with tools to track your progress.

If you've experienced positive results from the Great Physician's Rx for Diabetes program, I encourage you to reach out to others you know and recommend this book and program to them. You can learn how to lead a small group at your church or home by visiting www.GreatPhysiciansRx.com.

Remember: You don't have to be a doctor or a health expert to help transform the life of someone you care about—you just have to be willing.

Allow me to offer this prayer of blessing from Numbers 6:24–26 for you:

May the LORD bless you and keep you.

May the LORD make His face to shine upon you and be gracious unto you.

May the LORD lift up His countenance upon you and bring you peace.

In the name of Yeshua Ha Mashiach, Jesus our Messiah.

Amen.

Need Recipes?

For a detailed list of more than two hundred healthy and delicious recipes contained in the Great Physician's Rx eating plan, please visit www.GreatPhysiciansRx.com.

NOTES

Introduction

1. Jeffrey Krasner, "Diabetes Therapy Deal," *Boston Globe*, 16 March 2005.

Key #1

1. Lyle MacWilliam, "Diabetes: Understanding and Preventing the Next Health Care Epidemic," *LifeExtension*, June 2004.

2. "Consumer Group Wants Health Warnings on Soft Drinks," ConsumerAffairs.com, July 14, 2005.

3. Associated Press, "Study: Soda May Increase Diabetes Risk for Women," *USA Today*, June 8, 2004.

4. "The Secret Dangers of Splenda (Sucralose), an Artificial Sweetener," mercola.com, http://www.mercola.com/2000/dec/3/sucralose_dangers.htm#.

5. F. Batmanghelidj, M.D., *You're Not Sick, You're Thirsty!* (New York: Warner Books, 2003), 225–26.

6. Dr. Isadore Rosenfield, "Big News About a Little Spice," *Parade*, June 13, 2004.

Key #2

1. T. A. Barringer, J. K. Kirk, A. C. Santaniello, *et al.*, "Effect of a Multivitamin and Mineral Supplement on Infection and Quality of Life," *Annals of Internal Medicine*, March 3, 2003, 365–71.

2. "Fish Oil Lowers Triglycerides with Little or No Glycemic Effect in Type 2 Diabetics," *Reuters Health*, October 2005, http://www.diabeteslibrary.org/news/news_item.cfm?NewsID=229.

Key #3
1. "Diabetes Forum," manned by the staff at Gopi Memorial Hospital in Salem Tamilnadu, India, http://www.diabetesforum.net/eng_treatment_personalHygiene.htm.

Key #4
1. Randy Dotinga, "Too Little Sleep Could Cause Diabetes," *HealthDay*, April 27, 2005, http://health.yahoo.com/news/61350.

2. Nanci Hellmich, "Sleep Loss May Equal Weight Gain," *USA Today*, December 6, 2004, http://www.usatoday.com/news/health/2004-12-06-sleep-weight-gain_x.htm.

Key #5
1. Don Colbert, M.D., *Toxic Relief* (Lake Mary, FL: Siloam, 2003), 15.

2. F. Batmanghelidj, M.D., *You're Not Sick, You're Thirsty!* (New York: Warner, 2003), 2–3.

Key #6
1. Laurent C. Brown, BSCPHARM, Sumit R. Majumdar, MD, MPH, FRCPC, Stephen C. Newman, MD, MA, MSC, and Jeffrey A. Johnson, PHD, "History of Depression Increases Risk of Type 2 Diabetes in Younger Adults," *Diabetes Care* 28:1063–1067, 2005.

ABOUT THE AUTHORS

Jordan Rubin has dedicated his life to transforming the health of others one life at a time. He is a certified nutritional consultant, a certified personal fitness instructor, a certified nutrition specialist, and a member of the National Academy of Sports Medicine.

Mr. Rubin is the founder and chairman of Garden of Life, Inc., a health and wellness company based in West Palm Beach, Florida, that produces whole food nutritional supplements and personal care products. He is also president and CEO of GPRx, Inc., a biblically based health and wellness company providing educational resources, small group curriculum, functional foods, nutritional supplements, and wellness services.

He and his wife, Nicki, married in 1999 and are the parents of a toddler-aged son, Joshua. They make their home in Palm Beach Gardens, Florida.

Joseph D. Brasco, M.D., who is board certified in internal medicine and gastroenterology, is in private practice in Indianapolis, Indiana. He has skillfully combined diet, supplementation, and judicious use of medications to provide a comprehensive and effective treatment program. Dr. Brasco is the coauthor of *Restoring Your Digestive Health* with Jordan Rubin.

The Great Physician's Rx DVD and Study Guide

LEARN AND APPLY 7 TIPS TO GOOD HEALTH

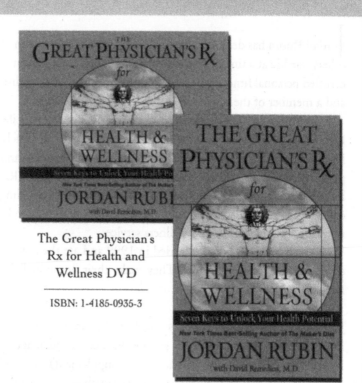

The Great Physician's
Rx for Health and
Wellness DVD

ISBN: 1-4185-0935-3

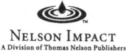

NELSON IMPACT
A Division of Thomas Nelson Publishers
Since 1798

www.thomasnelson.com

The Great Physician's
Rx for Health and
Wellness Study Guide

ISBN: 1-4185-0934-5

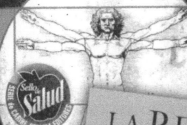

The Great
Physician's RX
available in Spanish

Sello de
Salud
SELLO DE CARIBE-BETANIA EDITORES

LA RECETA DEL
GRAN MÉDICO

para

TENER SALUD Y
BIENESTAR
EXTRAORDINARIOS

Siete claves para descubrir el potencial de su salud

Autor de un éxito de librería del New York Times

JORDAN RUBIN

y David Remedios, M.D.

CARIBE-BETANIA EDITORES
Una división de Thomas Nelson Publishers
www.caribebetania.com

ISBN: 0881130657

BHI

BIBLICAL HEALTH
INSTITUTE

The Biblical Health Institute (www.BiblicalHealthInstitute.com) is an online learning community housing educational resources and curricula reinforcing and expanding on Jordan Rubin's Biblical Health message.

Biblical Health Institute provides:

1. "101" level **FREE**, introductory courses corresponding to Jordan's book The Great Physician's Rx for Health and Wellness and its seven keys. Current "101" courses include:

   * "Eating to Live 101"

   * "Whole Food Nutrition Supplements 101"

   * "Advanced Hygiene 101"

   * "Exercise and Body Therapies 101"

   * "Reducing Toxins 101"

   * "Emotional Health 101"

   * "Prayer and Purpose 101"

2. **FREE** resources (healthy recipes, what to E.A.T., resource guide)

3. **FREE** media—videos and video clips of Jordan, music therapy samples, etc.—and much more!

Additionally, Biblical Health Institute also offers in-depth courses for those who want to go deeper.

Course offerings include:

   * 40-hour certificate program to become a Biblical Health Coach

   * A la carte course offerings designed for personal study and growth

   * Home school courses developed by Christian educators, supporting home-schooled students and their parents (designed for middle school and high school ages)

For more information and updates on these and other resources go to
www.BiblicalHealthInstitute.com

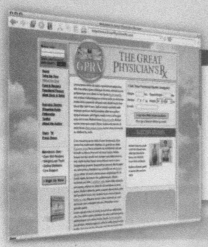

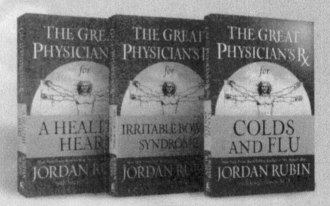

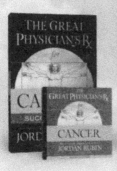
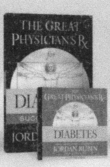
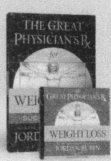